Handbook of Traction, Casting and Splinting Techniques

Handbook of Traction, Casting and Splinting Techniques

Royce C. Lewis, Jr., M.D.

Associate Clinical Professor of Orthopedic Surgery
and Director, Hand Surgery Service
Texas Tech University School of Medicine
Lubbock, Texas

J. B. Lippincott Company

Philadelphia · Toronto

ISBN 0-397-50380-6

Library of Congress Catalog Card Number 77-10326

Printed in the United States of America

6 5 4 3 2

Library of Congress Cataloging in Publication Data

Lewis, Royce C
Handbook of traction, casting and splinting techniques.

Includes index.
1. Orthopedic traction. 2. Plaster casts, Surgical.
3. Splints (Surgery) I. Title.
RD736.T7L48 617'.1 77-10326
ISBN 0-397-50380-6

Preface

Since prehistoric times it has been recognized that fractures, particularly of the long bones of the extremities, often require a longitudinal pull along the long axis of the extremity in order to reestablish alignment. On these early primitive efforts at realignment of long-bone fractures there has gradually developed a rather elaborate and sophisticated collection of traction techniques which have become well established as appropriate treatment for many fractures in the skeleton. The development of most of these techniques has occurred during the 19th and 20th centuries, with early orthopaedists using traction techniques almost exclusively in treatment of fractures. With newer surgical techniques there has been a considerable swing to open reduction in the treatment of many types of fractures. However, there are still many fractures that are best treated by continuous traction, and almost all fractures in the body *can* be treated by this method if the surgeon desires.

Since these traction techniques have been developed over a period of many years by a great many very inventive men, a multitude of traction techniques has been reported. As varied as these techniques may be they still must be based on certain specific principles if they are to be successful. By the same token, strict adherence to these principles of traction application will yield almost universally good results if the appropriate indications are present for their use.

It is the purpose of the section on traction techniques to establish a classification and description of these various principles of traction application. It is further hoped that by identifying these principles as such and by demonstrating how much the popular techniques in use today depend upon these specific principles the understanding of traction techniques will become much easier. If this section of the book can help establish some order out of the chaos that has developed in the minds of many people concerning traction techniques in general, it has served its purpose well.

Just as traction procedures have provided the mechanism for reducing and maintaining fractures in position while healing occurs, casting with rigid plaster-of-paris bandages has provided a mechanism for holding fractures in position once reduction has been achieved by some other mechanism. Probably no other discovery in the history of the treatment of musculoskeletal conditions has improved the effectiveness of immobilization as much as the use of rigid circumferential casts applied to the torso and extremities. Plaster casts or splints have provided the practitioner with close-fitting, efficient, and strong appliances for holding the bones or joints in almost any position desired.

It is this ability to effectively immobilize the musculoskeletal system that has made it possible for many fracture patients to be ambulatory who would otherwise have required protracted periods of immobility in traction, to hold the part in proper position for the long weeks often necessary for healing to occur.

As the art has developed, it has become apparent that while dynamic reduction of fractures or deformities is seldom possible with rigid plaster bandages, immobilization, per se, is often accomplished much more effectively with these appliances than with traction. While it is true that certain types of casts or splints can be developed that have a dynamic corrective force, the primary use of these devices is usually that of passive holding of the extremity in a predetermined position.

With these basic concepts in mind, then, one can explore the more sophisticated variations that have been developed over the years as plaster and other rigid materials have been refined technically and as the skill of physicians treating these musculoskeletal maladies has improved.

It is the purpose of the section on Cast and Splinting Techniques to develop these concepts in light of the volume of present knowledge and expertise available in medicine today. No effort has been made to discuss every situation requiring immobilization with rigid dressings or correction with dynamic splinting. Rather, an attempt has been made to define broad concepts and to develop in the reader a "feel" for the use of these appliances that should make it possible for him not only to apply these standard and "classic" cast models properly, but to be able to use personal creativity and ingenuity in his approach to specific problems encountered in everyday practice. If this type of judgement can be imparted, much will have been accomplished.

Royce C. Lewis, Jr.

Contents

Handbook of Traction, Casting and Splinting Techniques

1 Traction—General Considerations

PURPOSE OF TRACTION

When one begins a study of the various techniques of traction, the discussion should begin with the basic objective of traction in the treatment of fractures. In this way, one can more easily understand why traction is successful when properly applied. It can be most simply stated that traction is a mechanism by which the mechanical factors responsible for deformity in fractures of the long bones can be overcome, and alignment restored. A further development of this concept makes it important to consider the primary factors that result in deformity following loss of continuity of a portion of the skeleton. These factors are: (1) the mechanical force that resulted in the fracture occurring in the first place, (2) the effect of muscle tone, and (3) the effect of gravity. It is the sum of these three factors that results in displacement of the bone fragments once continuity has been lost, each occurring to a greater or lesser degree in a specific fracture and a specific circumstance.

Conversely, the overcoming of these three factors by the application of traction results in restoration of normal alignment. An analysis of these factors individually is important if one is to understand their significance in successful use of traction.

Overcoming the Deforming Effect of Force

The fracture of a bone, particularly one of the long bones of an extremity, generally occurs when force is applied to it in increasing amounts until it overcomes the structural stability of the bone. Even though this application of force often occurs suddenly, so that its effect seems almost instantaneous, a careful analysis reveals that the force usually is increased in a crescendo manner until a given amount suddenly causes a disruption of the continuity of the bone. In most instances, it is not possible to suddenly negate this force as soon as the bone breaks. The force itself carries through to result in increasing loss of position of the fragments, once disruption has occurred. Occasionally, the force is barely enough to produce a fracture; the force is spent almost by the time that fracturing occurs. There is not enough residual force left to result in displacement of the fragments. In fact, many times the fracture occurs as an incomplete crack through the bone or a fracture through the bone substance, with position being maintained by intact periosteum and soft tissue. These fractures are not included in this discussion. Fractures that are caused by a force in excess of the amount required to disrupt the continuity of the bone are important here. In these fractures, the force carries the fragments a variable distance from the normal alignment before it is negated. There is not sufficient counterforce to restore those bones to their normal alignment, and displacement of the fragments persists. In some cases, the force is so great that actual tearing of the soft tissue occurs. Occasionally, disruption of soft tissue may occur, which results in traumatic amputation of the part. In most instances, however, it is the soft tissue that constitutes the limiting factor to displacement. There results a soft-tissue compartment within which the fragments are retained.

The application of longitudinal traction, as shown in Figure 1-1, will result in realignment of these fractures by causing a molding of the fragments within the soft-tissue tube or compartment. Reapposition of the fragments is not possible when there is interposition of soft tissue between the fragment ends. The application of longitudinal pull will result in realignment of the soft-tissue structures along their original lines, as well as a reestablishment of original alignment of the bony structures. Since there already has occurred a cessation of the original deforming force, these structures can be maintained in their normal alignment by maintenance of traction. It should be pointed out that occasionally the deforming force may be related to gravity; it is the weight of the body applied transversely across the longitudinal axis of the bone that results in fractures sustained in a fall. However, the gravity itself is to be considered a deforming force, since its effect is still present even after the fracture has occurred. Once the body is no longer in a kinetic relationship to the ground, the original force that resulted in the fracture is also no longer present. In these instances, the implications for traction are the same as with other forces resulting in fractures.

Overcoming the Effect of Gravity

Following fractures, the continuing effect of gravity as a deforming factor occurs almost always in the case of long-bone fractures. It results from a bowing at the fracture site as the extremity is held in a horizontal position with relative support at either end of the bone. Gravity also has some effect in creating deformity following fractures in which the weight of the body superior to the fracture, no matter what its attitude, is great enough to result in a collapse or telescoping of the fracture. In either event, the application of traction results in an overcoming of the effect of gravity. Whether the weight of the body superior to the fracture is lifted off by this traction, counteracting the effect of gravity, or whether the effect is bowing in mid-shaft fractures held horizontally, the same principle is applied. The application of suitable pull along the long axis of the bone either lifts off the deforming "weight," or counteracts vectored force of gravity which causes bowing at the fracture site. Normal alignment is restored. Once the static effect of gravity is counteracted, the soft-tissue sleeve again molds the fracture site into normal anatomic position. These effects are demonstrated in Figure 1-2.

Overcoming the Effect of Muscle Pull

Fractures in an extremity with flaccid paralysis sometimes go unnoticed because they exhibit few deformities. The lack of displacement in the extremity with no nerve supply is due to the absence of muscle tone. Normal muscles exhibit a certain amount of contractive activity even at rest; it is this normal

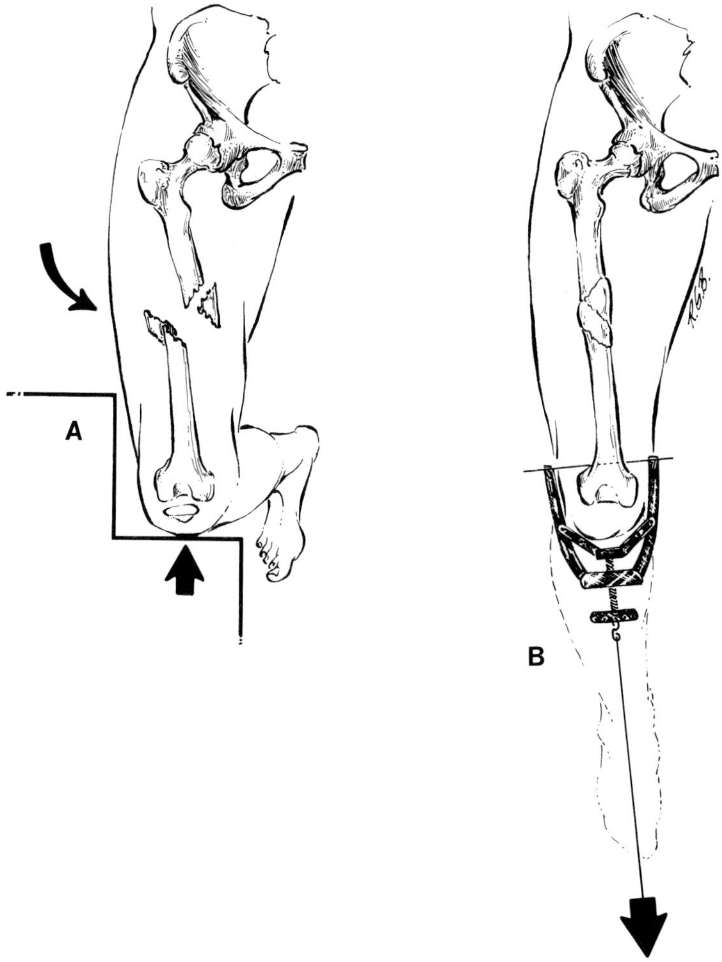

Fig. 1-1. The force that originally resulted in a fracture is one of the factors that causes deformity at the site of fracture. *(A)* The effect of force in a fracture of the femur. The weight of the body produces telescoping and angulation at the fracture site. The counterforce at the knee results in the formation of a relatively stable segment. The mobile segment is the proximal femoral fragment, and the remainder of the body acts under the force of gravity. *(B)* The effect of traction in overcoming the deforming force. Here, the body acts as a stable segment, and the longitudinal pull along the long axis of the femur has restored the normal alignment. The soft-tissue sleeve that is formed by the musculature around the fracture site has been drawn tightly by the traction, molding the smaller butterfly fragments into position.

tone, plus the added power of muscle spasm caused by the injury, that results in displacement of the fracture. The mechanics of muscle action dictate that the belly of the muscle lie over the shaft of the bone and that each end be attached at or near the ends of the bone. Loss of structural stability in the shaft of the bone allows the muscle to angulate or cause over-riding at the fracture site, as shown in Figure 1-3. This probably is the most consistent and the most important cause of persistent deformity in long bone fractures. It would follow, therefore, that overcoming this force by traction along the long axis of the

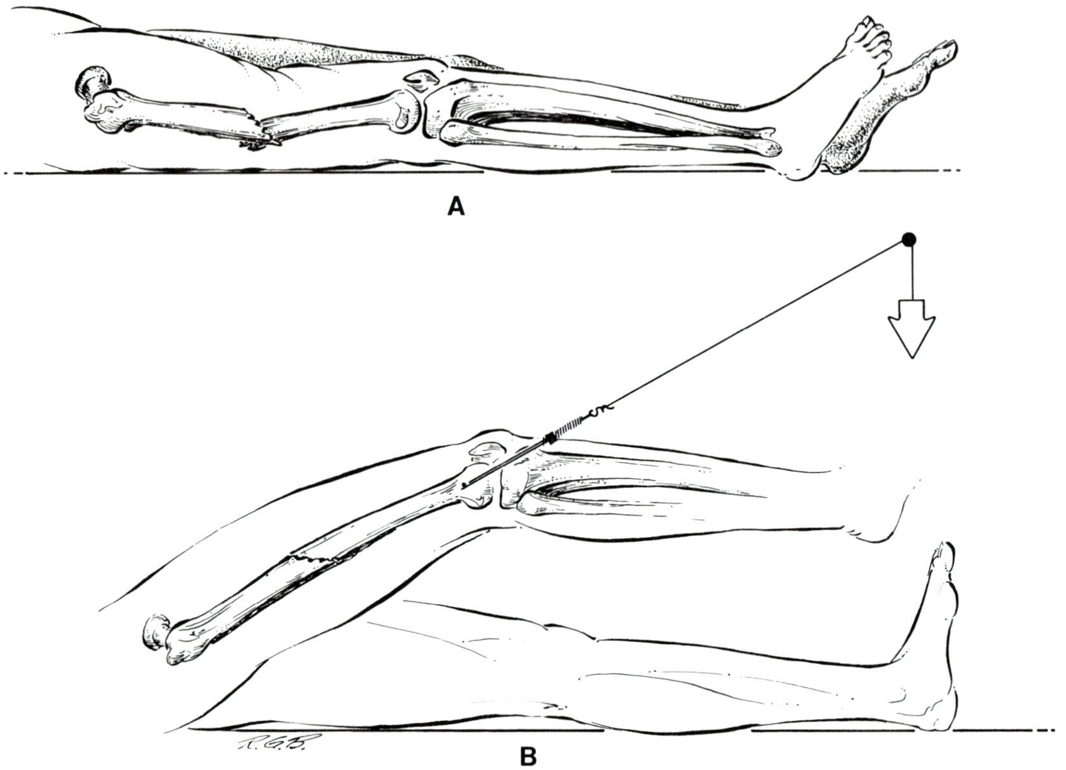

Fig. 1-2. (A) Posterior bowing at the site of fracture of the mid-femur. The body and the extremity distal to the fragment act as more-or-less fixed segments, so that the effect of gravity results in a bowing at the unstable fracture site. *(B)* The effect of traction in overcoming the force of gravity. As traction is applied along the longitudinal axis of the femur, the effect of gravity is overcome and the soft-tissue compartment is stretched so that it becomes tight. It acts as a molding force around the fracture.

muscle belly, in an amount slightly greater than the force of muscle pull, will allow a restoration of the normal structural position. This is true even when multiple fragments exist, with the muscle again forming a soft tissue tube that "molds" the fragments into place.

A word of caution is necessary concerning the tendency to overpull. It is imperative that the muscle pull *only* be overcome, and that enough "tone" be left in the muscles to hold the bone ends together for subsequent healing. If a greater force is used, the normal effect of muscle in holding the fracture ends in apposition is overcome, and distraction may occur. This results not only in a delayed healing or an occasional prevention of union, but also when healing *does* occur, the extremity may be lengthened. This is especially true in children who have elastic soft-tissue structures. Such overpull may result in lengthening of an extremity by several centimeters, with accompanying disability or functional loss. It is the overcoming of these various deforming forces, then, that constitutes the basis for effective use of traction in treating long-bone fractures.

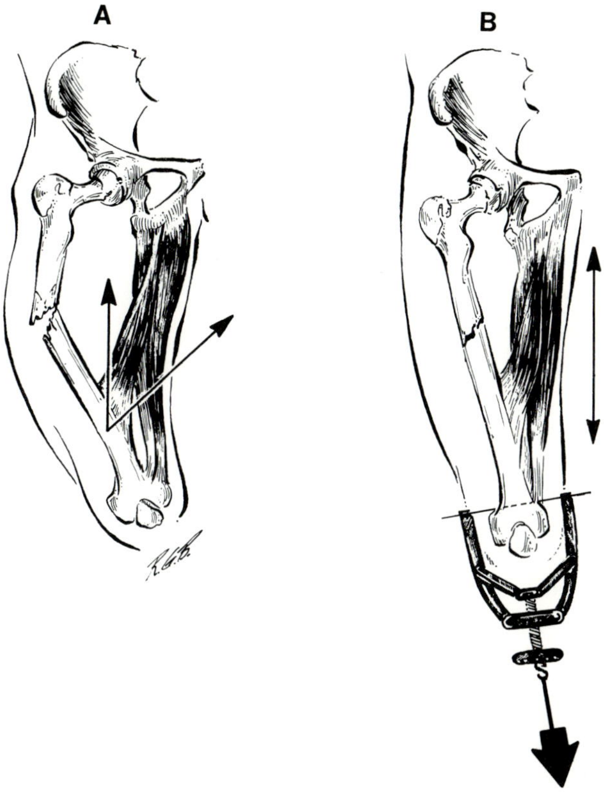

Fig. 1-3. One of the greatest deforming factors in fractures of the long bones is muscle pull. *(A)* A fracture at the mid-point of the femoral shaft is deformed in a lateral bow by the effect of tight adductor musculature. The adductors have the mechanical advantage, since they do not run exactly parallel with the long bone, as does the vastus lateralis on the lateral side. The musculature acts in a contracting manner to draw the two ends of the long bone closer together, resulting in lateral bowing. *(B)* The overcoming of muscle pull by traction. The muscles are stretched and their spasticity is overcome by the traction. The deforming bowstringing effect is counteracted and the femoral-shaft fracture assumes its normal anatomic alignment once the deforming factor is negated.

HOW MUCH TRACTION?

While one considers the amount of traction that is necessary, it becomes obvious that one must also consider the deforming factor that is to be overcome. As mentioned, the force of injury itself usually is momentary, and does not constitute a deforming force. This, therefore, leaves us with two primary deforming factors that must be overcome, namely, muscle pull and the effect of gravity. Of these two, the more important is the effect of muscle pull.

The Effect of Muscle Pull

In most instances, it is the overcoming of muscle pull that is the primary objective in treatment with traction. It would follow that the amount of traction necessary is related to the type of muscles surrounding the fracture site. In the heavily muscled individual this will require a much greater amount of traction; contrariwise, in the frail or smaller individual, the amount will be much less. The same is true with regard to the extremity involved. Fracture of the femur, for instance, requires much greater traction than fracture of the humerus in the same individual, since the surrounding musculature is much greater. It is extremely important when adjusting the traction to try to regulate the amount of weight, so that the effect of these deforming features is just overcome, but not unduly so. The overapplication of weight results in a distraction of the fragments, delayed healing, or failure to heal entirely. The effect of gravity usually is a much less important force than that of the deforming muscle pull. For this reason, as a general rule, if the amount of weight is great enough to overcome the muscle pull, *per se*, then the effects of gravity are automatically overcome. This is not invariably true, however, in instances in which relatively weak musculature exists around the fracture site.

The Effect of Gravity

Many times, the pull of gravity will result in a bowing of the fracture at the fracture site, even though the muscle pull has been satisfactorily overcome. The effect of gravity may be compensated by the application of an additional traction strap at the apex of the fracture to give a more direct pull against gravity. This is demonstrated in Figure 1-4. It is also possible to overcome the less deforming effect of gravity by placing the extremity in some sort of carrier, such as a Thomas traction setup, and perhaps by adding a small pad underneath the apex of the fracture to give additional support against the effect of gravity. Finally, the use of the so-called 90-90 traction in children is designed specifically to overcome this effect. By making the pull on the fracture at right angles to the pull of gravity, the deforming effect of gravity in creating angulation at the fracture site is obviated. The effect of gravity and the effect on muscle pull, therefore, are combined in a single plane which may be overcome by traction in a single direction. This is much easier to control since a single pull is necessary. The effect of gravity, then, is important only when its pull is not in the same direction as the deforming effect of muscle pull.

Fig. 1-4. (Opposite) Traction overcoming a composite deforming force composed of the effect of gravity and the effect of muscle pull, acting simultaneously. *(A,1)* The effect of gravity is shown as being present, even though the effect of muscle pull is overcome by longitudinal traction. *(A,2)* A sling has been added at the point of bowing of the fracture. The pressure of the sling and the longitudinal pull along the long axis of the femur have restored normal position of the fragments. *(A,3)* The sling under the bowed segment of femur has been replaced by a pad that mechanically lifts up the portion of the bone bowed by the effect of gravity. This, along with longitudinal pull, results in resumption of normal anatomic alignment. *(B)* Both of these factors can be overcome simultaneously. The traction is placed with the hip and knee at 90 degrees of flexion. The traction is placed on the femur; in this position the effect of muscle pull and of gravity, represented by weight of the distal fragment and leg, is overcome by the traction. The bowing effect of gravity is overcome, since the long axis of the femur is placed parallel to the pull of gravity; the bowing effect is negated and the fracture is held in anatomic alignment by the pull of the traction.

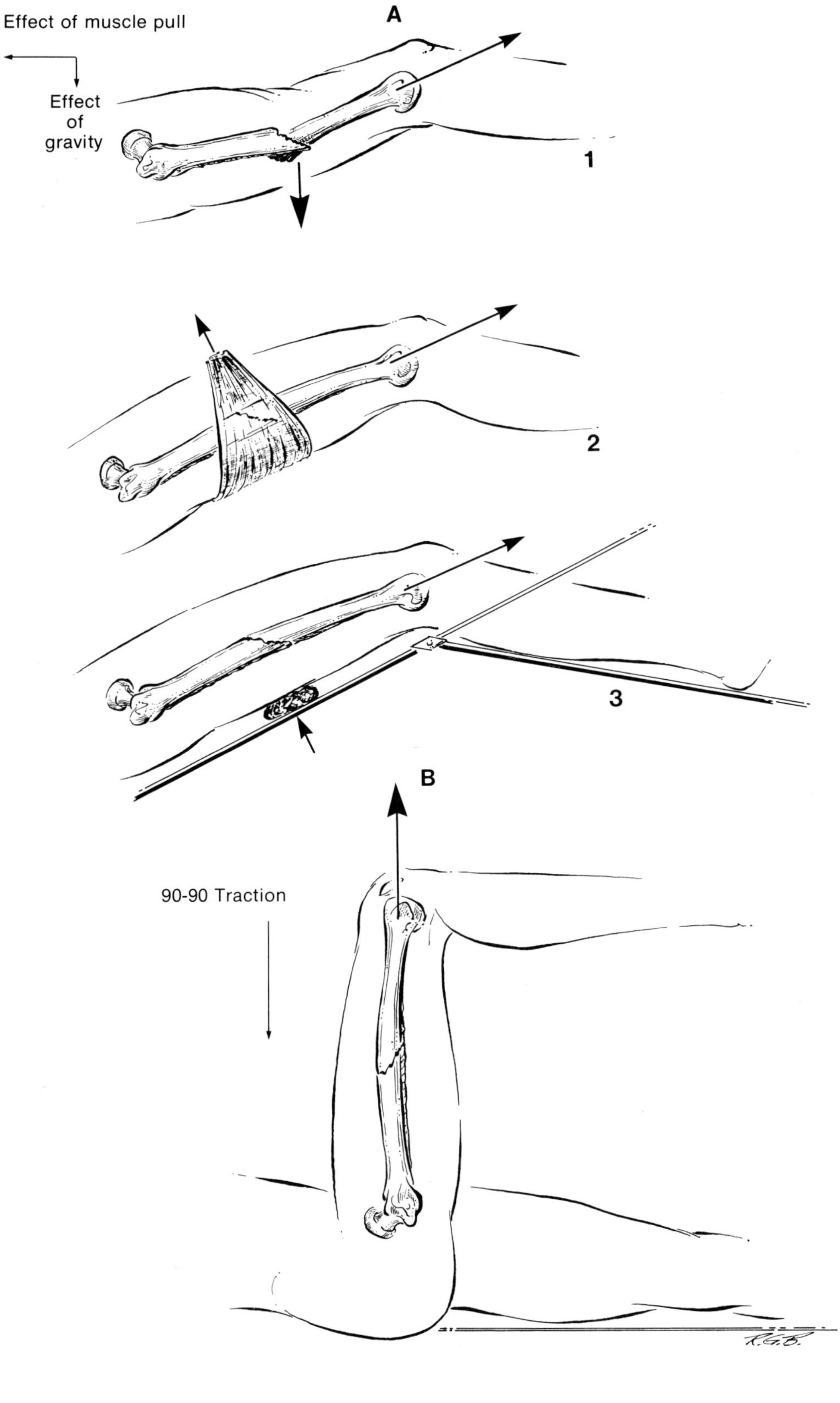
A
Effect of muscle pull
Effect of gravity
1
2
3
B
90-90 Traction
R.G.B.

General Considerations

The importance of serial x-ray examinations cannot be overemphasized; it is only by monitoring the position of the fracture by roentgenograms that satisfactory results can be obtained. It is very important in the early stages of treatment of fractures by traction to check the position and effect of traction often by portable roentgenograms.

The addition or subtraction of traction in this stage often will result in the direct change in the position of the fragments. However, as time goes on, and early healing occurs at the fracture site, the addition and subtraction of weight on the traction apparatus is much less likely to have any dramatic effect; errors in the amount of traction applied are much more likely to produce permanent problems.

The amount of traction will dictate the mechanism of attachment of the traction apparatus to the extremity. This is discussed in greater detail in Chapter 2. However, it should be pointed out that if the necessary amount of pull is great, skeletal attachment must be obtained with the use of traction pins. The skin and soft tissue are not able to withstand great amounts of traction. Damage to the skin will occur if one attempts to apply too great an amount of traction by skin attachment rather than by skeletal attachment utilizing a traction pin drilled through the bone. For instance, it is seldom possible to treat femoral fractures with skin traction, except in the very young. If the individual is of larger size, with musculature that is well developed, it is mandatory to use skeletal traction rather than relying on traction tapes or other fixation devices attached to the skin and soft tissue.

Fig. 1-5. (Opposite) (A) A fracture of the mid-shaft of the femur, which has had a traction pin inserted through the distal fragment, with longitudinal pull of a sufficient amount to reduce the fracture. As long as the extremity distal to the fracture site lies on the supporting surface or bed, two separate and distinct segments have been created: (1) The body segment is comprised of the body itself. The proximal fragment is immobile because the weight or pull of gravity is holding this segment to the bed. (2) The distal segment, consisting of that part of the extremity distal to the fracture site, is likewise relatively immobile because it lies on the bed. The pull of gravity or the weight of the extremity renders it relatively immobile. Motion occurs through the fracture site that lies between the two relatively immobile segments. *(B)* The extremity has been placed in a balanced suspension apparatus, so that the body segment is now that portion of the body that lies in contact with the bed. Now this segment ends at the buttocks or in the hip joint. By placing the entire extremity in a balanced setup so that it no longer comes in contact with the bed, but rather is suspended in a relatively weightless condition, the entire extremity has been transposed into a single segment that is relatively mobile. Any motion caused by movement of the patient's body or by swinging of the leg in the suspension apparatus will occur at the hip joint, since this represents the juncture between the two segments, as contrasted with the juncture in *(A)*, where movement occurs between the two segments at the fracture site. A balanced traction setup, therefore, not only reduces the fracture by longitudinal pull, but also immobilizes the fracture site by allowing motion to occur at the hip joint, rather than at the fracture site.

TYPES OF TRACTION

It is the purpose of this chapter to discuss traction, not from the standpoint of *specific* types, but rather to discuss the various *conceptual* types. The various principles of traction have been discussed previously. It now becomes proper to discuss the utilization of various forces to achieve the desired result, as described previously. When one considers the various types of traction, there appear to be three basic concepts that are in general use today: (1) straight traction, (2) so-called balanced traction, and (3) vectored traction.

Straight Traction

Straight traction, as the name implies, results basically in the application of some mechanism to create a pull on a portion of the body. This will, of course,

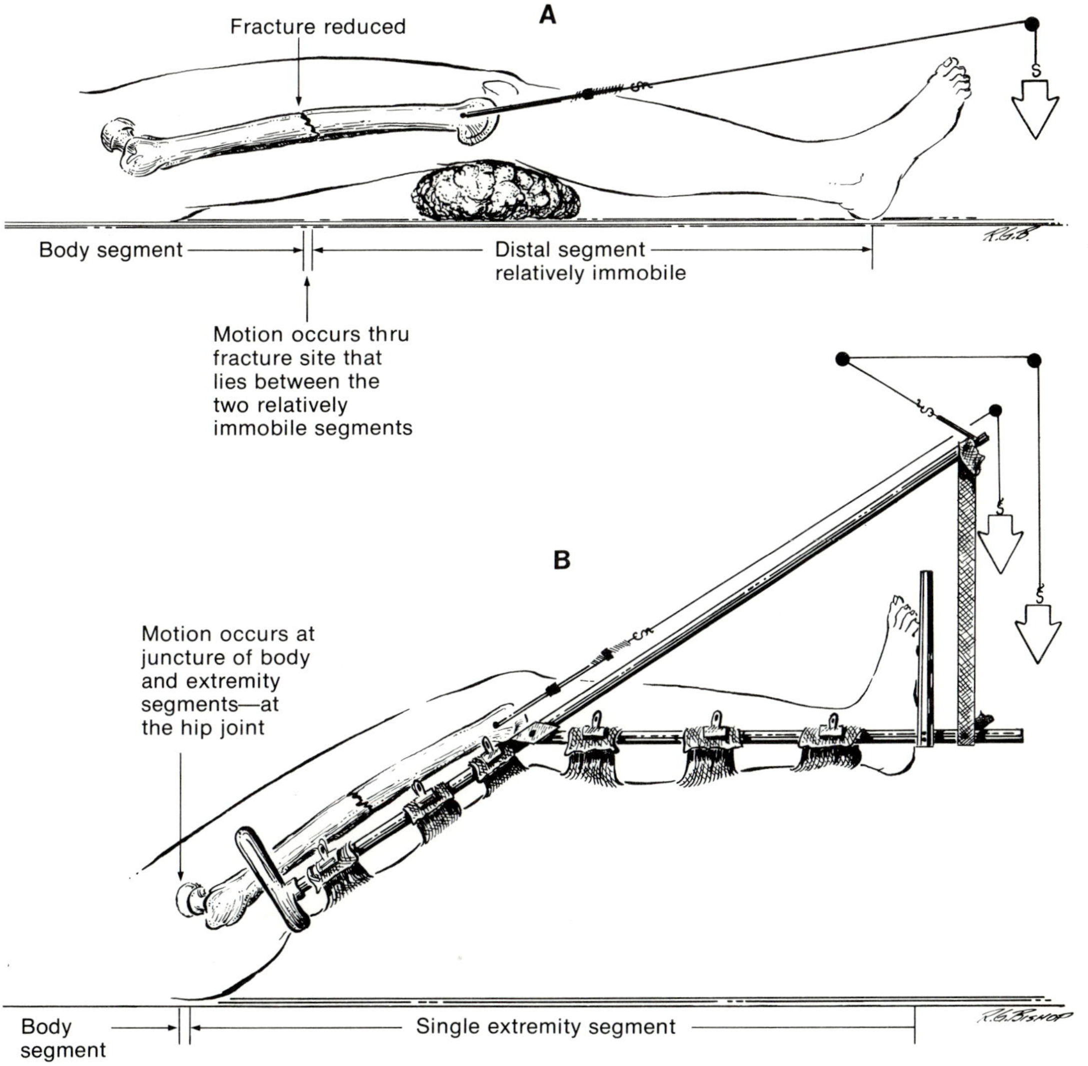

include Buck's traction in which, by applying traction either with tapes, foam strips, or a traction boot, there occurs a pull along the direct line of the extremity. This pull usually is of minimal force. It is not possible to apply a great amount of pull when skin traction is used, because it results in damage to the soft tissue.

Buck's traction is used for holding an extremity that has been injured, often while awaiting more definitive treatment. Traction of this nature will maintain the position of the fragments reasonably well and will help to overcome the effect of muscle spasm. Buck's traction also is used for immobilization of the lower extremity, such as after reduction of hip dislocations. It is used on some occasions for the application of traction to an extremity that is painful owing to nerve-root pressure in the lower back. In all of these instances, the traction is not important from the standpoint of definitive treatment. Most of the time, its application is principally a matter of attempting to maintain comfort.

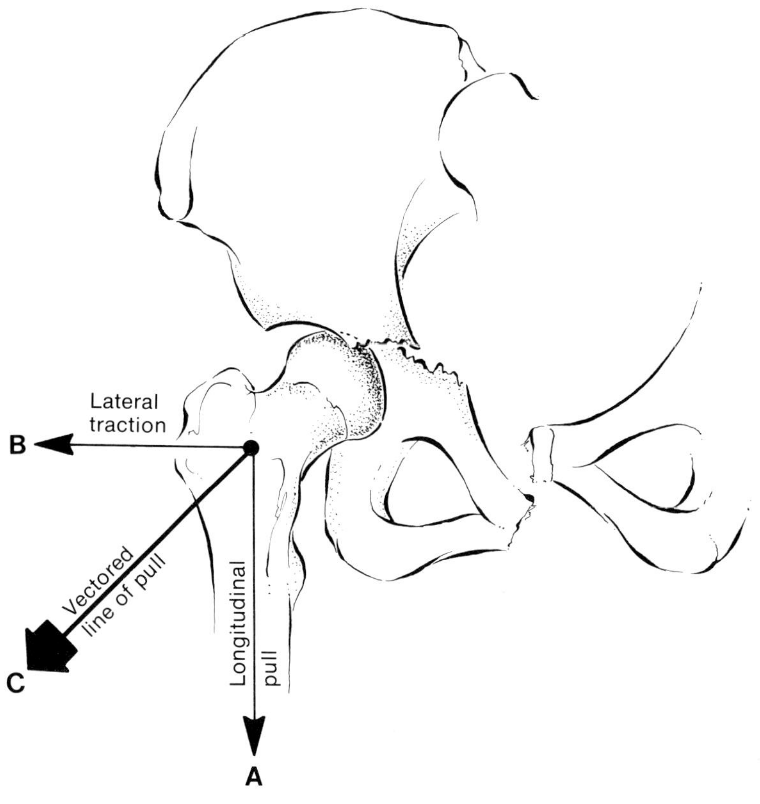

Fig. 1-6. An example of vectored traction is shown, in the case of a central fracture of the hip with intrapelvic protrusion of the femoral head. The line of traction that is desired is along the long axis of the femoral neck. Since it is very difficult to secure traction along this line, traction may be exerted at *B* by means of a trochanteric screw. Traction may then be supplied along *A* in a balanced traction setup, with a pin through the distal femur. The two forces of traction can be adjusted so that the effective line of traction may be vectored along a line somewhere in the vicinity of *C*.

Other types of straight traction are the pelvic traction that is used with disc syndromes in the low back, and halter traction used for disorders of the cervical spine and neck. Straight traction will also apply to the skeletal traction applied to the neck. This is a straight-line pull, even when it is applied through Crutchfield tongs or a halo apparatus attached to the skull for a skeletal traction. The principal pull is in a straight line without additional support or without additional traction in any other direction.

Balanced Traction

Balanced traction is probably the most common form of therapeutic traction used for definitive treatment of fractures and injuries to the extremities. The basic concept of balanced traction is that the extremity is suspended in some sort of a frame which holds the entire extremity and creates from the extremity a single "unit." For example, in the treatment of a fracture of the femur, if straight traction were applied, there would be extremely poor immobilization at the fracture site, even though the deforming factors of muscle pull would have been overcome and the fracture reduced. The extremity would lie on the bed and traction would be applied through the distal portion of the femur, perhaps through a skeletal pin, allowing for movement through the fracture site when any movement would occur in the body. In other words, the distal portion of the extremity, from the fracture down, would constitute a single segment that would be more or less immobilized by traction and by friction with the bed as its weight pressed the extremity against the bed. When motion occurred in the body, then, the most likely place of movement between the *body* segment and the distal extremity would be through the fracture site itself. A very poor form of immobilization would occur.

By suspending the extremity in a traction frame, such as a Thomas traction apparatus with Pierson attachment, and by counterbalancing it with weights, a more or less weightless condition is created. The entire extremity is transformed into a single segment or unit. This is shown in Figure 1-5, where the entire extremity has been transformed into a single mobile segment, and the juncture between the "extremity segment" and the "body segment" occurs at the hip joint. Motion occurs here rather than at the fracture site. The pull that has been applied through the skeletal fixation pin relieves the muscle spasm and corrects the deformity. The suspension in the balanced traction frame allows the fracture to be more completely immobilized by removing these stresses from it. Balanced traction is probably one of the favorite mechanisms for treating fractures of the long bones of the extremity, particularly the femur, and to a lesser extent, the humerus.

Vectored Traction

Occasionally, it is not possible to apply traction in the direct line of pull that is necessary to reduce a fracture or a dislocation. In these instances, it is often possible to apply traction in two different directions, with the two lines of pull at close to right angles. The resultant force, or "vectored force," occurs somewhere between the two lines of force being applied. It can be adjusted so that it occurs in the direction that is necessary for definitive treatment of the skeletal injury. Examples of this are shown in Figure 1-6 and 1-7. In Figure 1-6, the central fracture dislocation of the hip requires a pull along the line represented by "C" to reduce the femoral head to its location, and perhaps to reduce the pelvic fracture at the same time. It is extremely difficult to achieve a pull in this direction. It is possible to achieve a straight-line pull of the long axis of the femur line "A" by application of a trochanteric screw, which allows a completely level traction along line "D." This results in vectored force along line "C"—the desirable direction for reduction of the fracture-dislocation.

It sometimes also is desirable, for convenience, to apply traction as shown in Figure 1-7, in directions not precisely required for reduction and maintenance of the fractured long bone. In Figure *7A*, traction is being applied along the long axis of a femoral fracture. The extremity is suspended in a suspension sling for the balanced traction effect. If, however, it becomes necessary to remove the suspension frame because of pressure or other "nursing care" causes, it is possible to supply traction as shown in Figure 1-*7B*,, wherein the pull along line "1" not only supplies a certain amount of traction of the long axis of the femur, but also allows for the suspension of the leg itself. Traction along the line "2" is required to make the vectored force or the effective line of pull along line "3." This results in a complete resumption of traction in a vectored line of pull required for treatment of the fractured femur, even though the two lines of pull, "1" and "2," are not in this particular direction. The use of vectored

Fig. 1-7. (Opposite) (A) The typical balanced traction setup for the lower extremity. The basic suspension unit is composed of some type of traction frame, such as the Thomas traction ring or one of the various modifications. To this is attached an out-rigger that can be moved up or down the long axis of the basic traction frame so that the length of the femur can be accommodated. This small out-rigger, then, allows for the support of the extremity below the knee. The distal portion of the out-rigger is attached to the distal end of the main frame by means of tape or straps (*inset*). These may be adjusted to allow for variations in the amount of flexion at the knee, but as a general rule, approximately 45 degrees of flexion is desirable and is most comfortable. The amount of flexion at the knee does not materially influence the traction that occurs through the distal femur, proximal to the knee joint itself. The frame is suspended by a rope *(1)* that is attached to the distal end of the frame and passed through a pulley. The pulley is placed proximally, in order to support the frame in the elevated position. The rope then runs to a distal pulley and over to a weight. The amount of weight is that just sufficient to create a weightless condition in the extremity, so that the frame, being precisely counterbalanced, will stay in almost any position in which it is placed. A second line is then attached to the traction bow *(2)* and is brought either over or under the distal portion of the main traction frame. It is attached to a single pulley bearing the amount of weight that is deemed desirable for traction to the femur. It should be noted that the two weights have entirely different responsibilities, that through line *(1)* having the function of supporting the frame against the pull of gravity, and that of *(2)* furnishing the actual traction through the femur. *(B)* An alternative method for support of the extremity in a balanced traction setup. The same traction pin is inserted through the distal femur, with the traction bow being attached to line *(1)*. The pull through the traction is directly upward and at about 45° to the long axis of the femur. The lower extremity has been suspended in either a short-leg plaster cast or a traction boot. The pull is applied along the long axis of the lower leg, again, at about 45° to the long axis of the femur *(2)*. The resulting vectored pull should be along the line *(3)* in the long axis of the shaft of the femur. In this instance, the traction itself acts as the suspending mechanism.

traction is necessary only occasionally. Many times, however, it has a very definite application in effective traction of long bone fractures.

It will be seen, in chapters dealing with specific traction procedures for specific fractures, that almost all methods of traction treatment are adaptations of one of these three fundamental concepts of traction application.

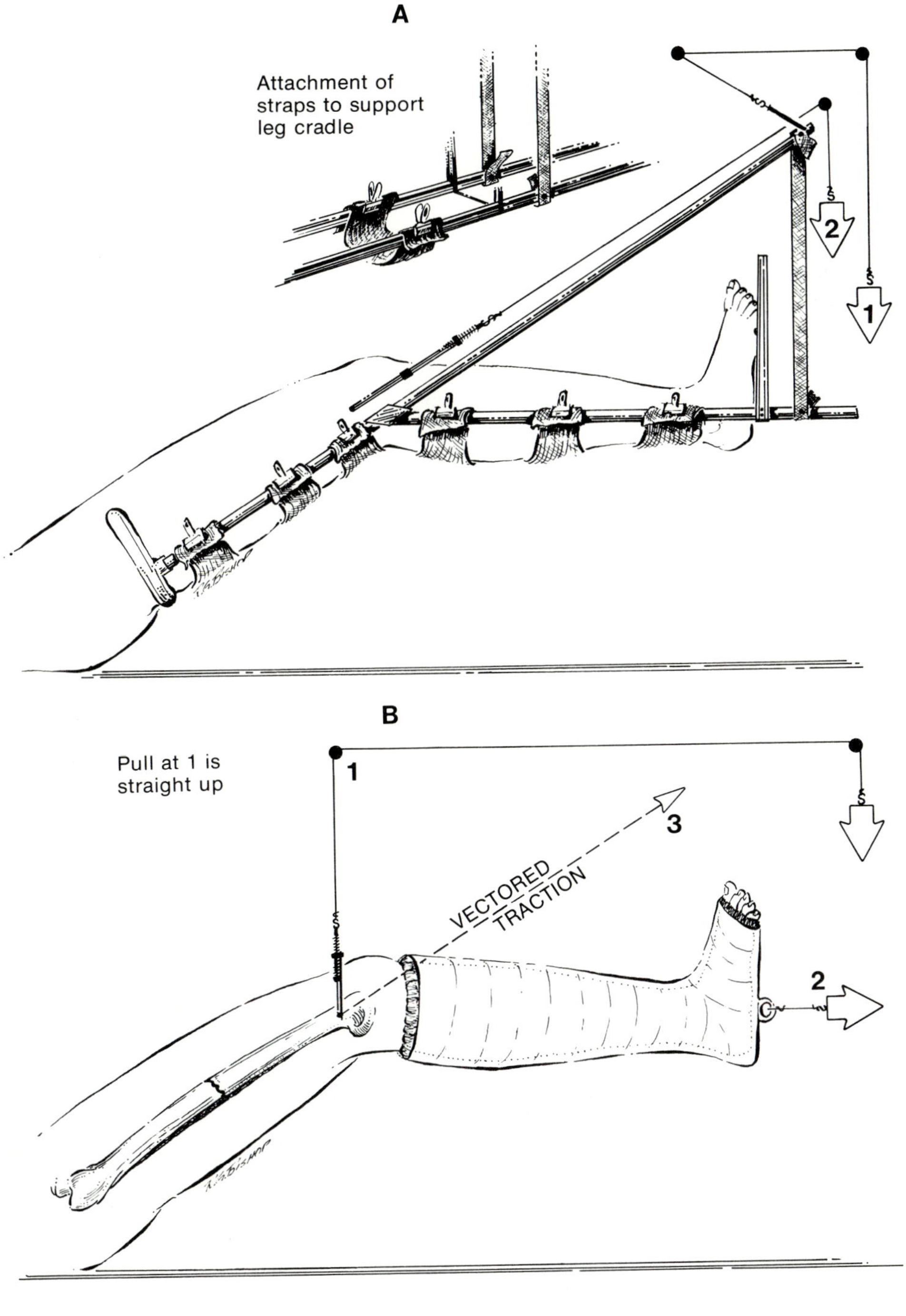

PULL THROUGH JOINTS

It is often necessary, in the course of application of traction to the extremity, to apply the pin at a point distal to the fracture. A joint may separate the site of the pin application from the fracture, resulting in a pull through the joint. This occurs, for instance, in supracondylar fractures of the humerus wherein a pin is drilled through the olecranon so that a longitudinal pull can be placed on the distal humerus. This results in a pull through the elbow joint, which seldom causes any real difficulty with the joint itself. Pull through other joints, however, occasionally does cause some difficulty. It is necessary, in some instances, to apply traction to the distal femur through a pin inserted through the upper tibia. This makes the line of pull different from that necessary for reduction of the fracture. However, if the knee is kept reasonably straight and particularly if a sling is added for a supportive power underneath the fracture itself (as shown in Figure 1-8*B*), the effect on the joint is not severe. When pull is of a considerable weight over a long period of time and the joint is in an unusual or strained position, then there occurs ligamentous damage to the joint, and irreparable changes can occur. Likewise, if the pin is placed too close to the joint, resulting in capsular edema and perhaps even in infection along the pin tract, serious complications can occur. If the traction is not great and the pin is placed so that the joint is not involved, traction can be placed through joints without serious difficulty.

In the case of a pin placed through the os calcis for traction on the distal tibia (pulling through the subastragalar and the ankle joints), the necessary pull can be maintained without harming the joints, provided the need for maintaining position is not great.

It goes without saying, however, that meticulous care of the pin tract must be carried out, particularly in those tracts adjacent to joints. Infection of the pin tract usually involves the joint directly; serious and permanent conse-

---

Fig. 1-8. (Opposite) Individual variations in the type of pull, the degree of pull, and the position of the associated joints. *(A)* Pull through the elbow joint by means of a pin attached to the olecranon for fractures of the distal humerus. These supracondylar fractures are more stable in flexion, but many times the elbow joint *per se* cannot be flexed past 90 degrees because of swelling in the antecubital space. The elbow joint may be maintained at 90 degrees by elevating the angle of the pull slightly, thus stabilizing the fracture and avoiding having to flex the elbow joint past 90°. *(B)* A fracture of the distal femur in an immature individual with open epiphyseal plates precludes the insertion of the traction pin in the femur. The traction pin is placed in the upper tibia, distal to its epiphyseal plate. The fracture is further stabilized by means of a sling underneath the distal femur, to prevent posterior bowing at the fracture site. The traction is still maintained in the line of the long axis of the femur and, with the addition of the supporting sling the reduction the reduction is maintained. *(C)* The effect of traction on the metacarpophalangeal joints of the hand. When traction is placed with this joint in extension, the collateral ligaments, which are at their shortened position in extension, may contract. There results loss of flexion in the joint. When traction is placed with the joint in flexion, which produces lengthening of the collateral ligaments, contracture of these ligaments is not possible. Flexion can be maintained after the discontinuation of the traction.

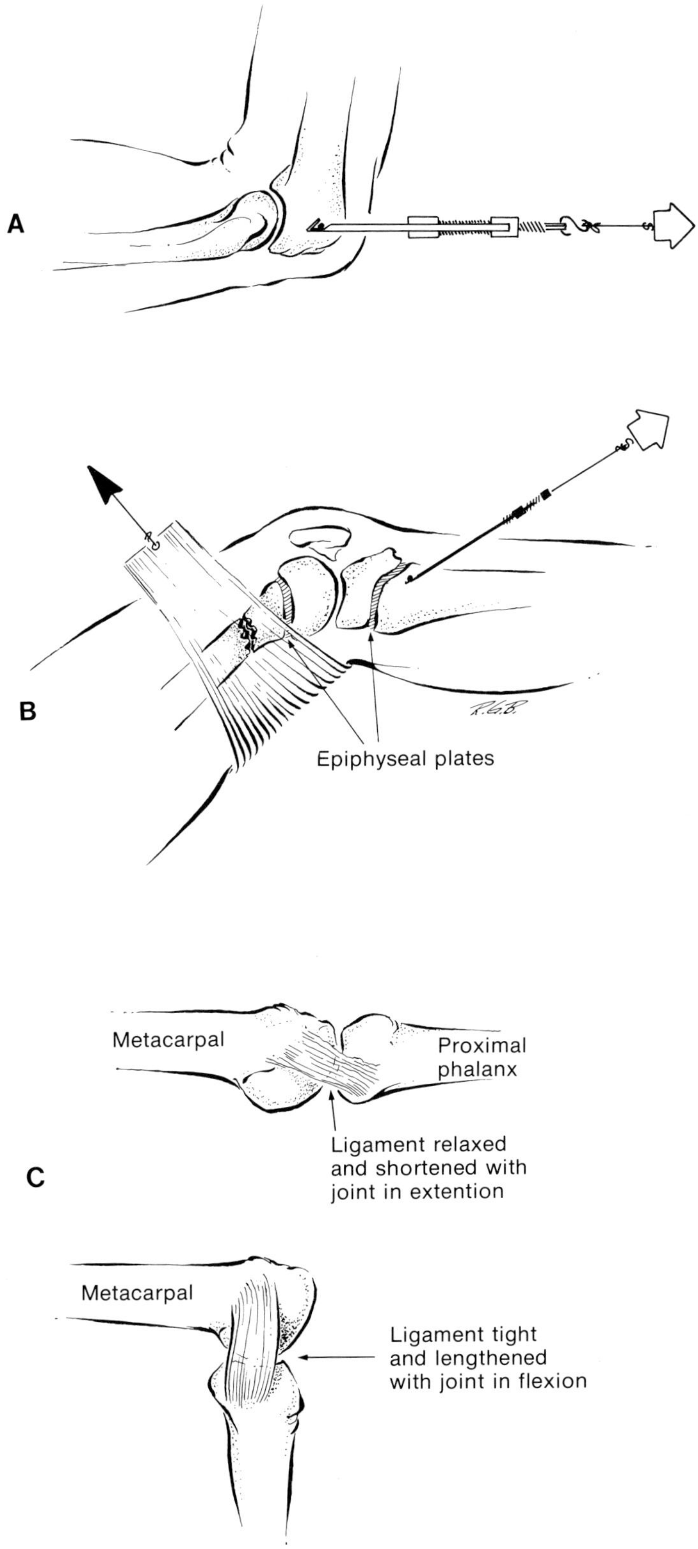
A
B
Epiphyseal plates
Metacarpal
Proximal phalanx
Ligament relaxed and shortened with joint in extention
C
Metacarpal
Ligament tight and lengthened with joint in flexion

quences can occur. Insertion of the pin in proper position, however, will often allow for traction where it would otherwise be impossible if the pin were not placed distal to the joint.

Traction of the Hands and Fingers

A special word should be made concerning traction to the joints of the hand. The old banjo traction apparatus, which applied traction in a straight line from the metacarpal shaft out to the distal phalanx, is mentioned only to vigorously condemn it. It has been shown that such traction often results in a very seriously damaged hand—damage occurring basically from the traction itself. Particularly in the case of the proximal joint of the fingers, the ligamentous attachments are such that the ligaments are in their longest position with the joint in 90 degrees of flexion. Contrariwise, with the joint in "0" degrees of extension, the ligamentous structures are relaxed. If the joint is pulled up in complete extension, particularly with traction to it, irreparable contractural changes occur in the ligamentous structures. The changes preclude regaining flexion in joints once the traction has been relieved. If the traction is to be placed on the fingers, care should be taken that the proximal and middle joints of the fingers are held in the position of flexion. The traction should be applied around a curve similar to the functional position of the hand. In no instance is it permissible to apply traction in a straight line with the joints all held in complete extension (Fig. 1-8*C*).

ATTACHMENT OF TRACTION TO AN EXTREMITY (SKIN VERSUS PIN)

The problem of attaching traction to an extremity concerns two possibilities, namely, skin traction versus pin traction. The decision as to which traction to use depends largely upon what is to be gained by the traction and the type of traction that is necessary. For instance, the skin traction, while much easier to apply than the pin traction, has limitations; the skin and soft tissue will tolerate only limited amounts of traction. It cannot be used when a great amount of muscle pull is to be overcome, or when a large amount of distraction is to be achieved. The fact that it can be applied without breaking the skin or entering the bone makes it much more desirable to use. Pin traction, on the other hand, does create problems that must be weighed against the advantages of its use.

Skin Traction

Skin Straps. When one speaks of skin traction there are actually three possibilities. Adhesive strips, mole skin, or thin sponge strips with multiple ventilation holes comprise the three presently used methods of skin attachment. These are demonstrated in Figure 1-9*A*. The straps may be either of adhesive mole skin or of sponge rubber, sponge rubber straps having the advantage of not requiring an adhesive to hold them to the skin. The adhesive strips and the mole skin, of course, necessitate the use of adhesive compound for attachment, which may result in blistering of the skin.

Also, adhesive strips often produce eruptions of the skin due to irritation

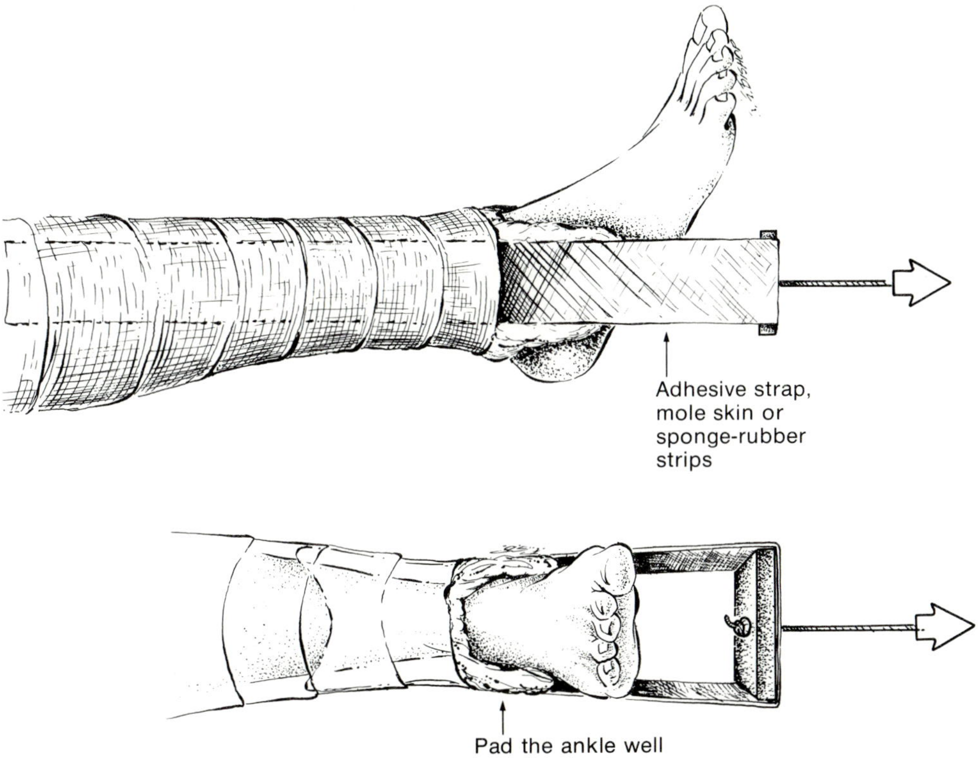

Fig. 1-9. Longitudinal traction of the lower extremity, such as Buck's traction, is accomplished by the use of straps made of adhesive mole skin or sponge-rubber-backed fabric strips. These adhere to the skin and are secured by circumferential wrapping, usually with elastic bandage. It is necessary to pad the ankle well, since these strips will cause pressure sores over the malleoli. A spreader bar or block is necessary to attach the traction rope to the strips so that they will pull in a longitudinal manner. A foam-rubber traction boot can also be used. (See Fig. 2-9.)

from the pull on the skin, as well as from the chemical irritation of the adhesive compound.

In all of these instances, it is necessary to wrap the extremity, usually with an elastic bandage, to hold the strips in place. Traction is applied over a spreader mechanism, which may either be a block or a metallic spreader made for that purpose. The traction, as mentioned, is limited in extent; great amounts of traction will result in such irritation of the skin that it cannot be tolerated over any period of time.

Foam Traction Boot. A newer addition to the appliances for application of skin traction is the foam traction boot. This boot is fashioned from relatively thick plastic sponge which is applied. (See Figure 1-9*B*.) The boot is held around the extremity with Velcro straps; the traction created between the foam plastic and the skin allows for a moderate amount of pull on the straps, which are positioned on either side and passed to a spreader block at the end. It is obvious, as with the preceding methods of skin traction, that only a moderate amount of traction will be tolerated because of the inability of the skin to sustain continuous irritation. In some instances, a boot cast can be used for moderate amounts of traction. This requires massive padding; traction on the longitudinal axis of a short-leg boot cast often results in pressure phenomena, particularly over the instep and heel. This method usually is not justified, particularly because the other methods are so readily available.

Pin Traction

Pin traction is by far the most practical method of applying great amounts of traction to the skeleton over a long period of time. The skin is aseptically prepared with scrubbing or antibacterial solutions, or both, and the pin is drilled through with either a mechanical drill or a small hand drill. A tiny opening is made in the skin with a sharp-pointed knife blade before the pin is introduced into the bone. It is then drilled through the bone and is allowed to emerge from the opposite side.

The pin itself may be one of two types. It may be a relatively large Steinmann pin, which is rigid enough to allow pull on its two sides by a simple horseshoe mechanism, without application of tension to the pin itself. However, the most widely used method is the insertion of a relatively small-gauge Kirschner wire with a traction bow apparatus applied to it. The traction bow grasps the wire on either side and stretches it tightly, making it quite rigid, so that traction can be applied through it. This allows for a much more substantial traction mechanism, and requires a much smaller opening in the skin and in the bone for insertion of the pin. Great amounts of traction can be applied to the long bones of the extremity through the Kirschner wire used in this manner. Usually, some type of antibacterial ointment is placed around the small openings in the skin where the pin protrudes. A dry dressing is applied over the pin site to protect the small wounds from secondary infection.

Advantages. The most obvious advantage is that traction can be applied directly to the skeleton without the interposition of soft tissue. This allows for a greater amount of traction, and allows it to be applied much more accurately. There are no skin problems present when pin traction is used, except for the possibility of infection around the pin site. Great amounts of weight can be applied to the skeleton, whereas with the skin traction it is difficult to apply more than 5 to 10 pounds for any length of time.

Complications. Pin tract infections occasionally occur and may lead to serious consequences. The infection seldom becomes severe enough to require removal of the pin; usually it can be kept under control by systemic antibiotics and local applications of heat. The total infectious process, however, cannot be completely eradicated until the foreign body (pin) is removed. When serious or uncontrollable infection does occur around the pin, it is advisable to remove the offending pin and insert another pin in a different location under stringent asepsis, so that the old infection will not be transferred.

A less common complication of pin traction is ring necrosis in bone around the pin site. This necrosis of bone may be related to the heat of friction as the pin is inserted. It also may result from infection occurring around the pin site, with sequestrum forming as a result of the infection. Many pin sites do have a certain amount of drainage, which results from irritation or foreign body reaction, and does not represent true pin-tract infection. Many times the pins become loose and slip from side to side. This inoculates the pin tract with bacteria each time it occurs, and constitutes a major problem in caring for the pin itself. In instances of pins slipping, thorough cleansing of the skin openings with hydrogen peroxide (3%) should be carried out daily, and antibiotic ointment should be applied. A pad can then be applied on either side to help stabilize the pin and prevent or minimize further slipping.

CARE OF TRACTION

This section is a final word concerning the general points of care in the use of traction. As has been mentioned previously, traction should not be used as a form of treatment unless arrangements are made for close supervision and daily adjustment. Well-conceived and well-planned traction requires constant supervision to be certain that the desired effect is being achieved. Many times it becomes necessary to alter the traction to secure proper alignment of the fracture fragments and to be certain that adequate traction is applied in the proper direction. These daily adjustments may be made by well-trained personnel other than the physician, but the physician, by use of periodic x-ray examination, must be certain that the proper ends have been achieved, and that proper alignment and position have been established and maintained with the traction. Aside from the possibility of malalignment and improperly applied traction, there are relatively few complications to traction therapy. Occasionally pressure sores develop. These usually are associated with the traction apparatus itself and are related to poor supervision. Occasionally pressure sores develop without being noticed and without patient complaint. At times, through no fault of the supervising personnel, a pressure sore will appear that has been unanticipated.

The patient will complain of a burning pain in the area that has undue pressure. These complaints should not be taken lightly; they should be investigated thoroughly to prevent pressure sores from developing. Pressure sores are extremely difficult to heal.They usually occur over structures that are best left covered and that become secondarily infected, with serious consequences to the surrounding vital structures.

Pin-tract drainage, as previously mentioned, is felt to be related to foreign-body reaction to the pin. Pin-tract infection can occur from inoculation of bacteria in the canal through which the pin passes; serious soft-tissue and bone infections may occur. At any indication that inflammatory signs are present around the pin tract, immediate measures should be instituted for management of the infection, including antibiotic therapy, warm compresses, and other standard treatments of local soft-tissue infection.

2 Specific Areas of Traction Application

With the general discussion of traction techniques in mind, it is necessary to discuss each of the specific areas of traction application. The types of traction vary greatly according to location and specific use in the body. While it is true that the basic principles are applicable no matter what part of the body is treated, the fact remains that specific areas have characteristics that differ from other parts of the musculoskeletal system. It is necessary to discuss each part separately in some detail.

CERVICAL SPINE

When it becomes necessary to apply traction to the cervical spine, the point of attachment of the traction device must be the cranium.

Halter Traction

For the vast majority of affectations of the cervical spine and neck, simple halter traction is sufficient to apply the amount of weight necessary. Cervical sprains, strains, and protruded cervical discs are all treated by halter traction applied with the patient lying supine in bed; the body itself supplies countertraction. As a general rule, the amount of traction that can be applied by halter is limited to not over 5 pounds. Often even this much weight is not tolerated for long periods of time. The halter, as demonstrated in Figure 2-1, impinges under the chin and under the occiput, and is fitted so that relatively even traction is applied to these two parts of the head.

Many physicians have preferences as to the line of pull that they feel is most advantageous in applying traction to the cervical spine. The fact that there is such a wide divergence of opinion as to the best position for traction makes it reasonable to believe that there is no single way that is superior. If the patient lies supine in bed with the head of the bed elevated approximately 30 to 35 degrees and the hips and knees flexed slightly, the hospital-bed traction can be administered in such a way that the line of pull extends all the way from the buttocks through the entire spine and head and through the rope into the pulley. From this neutral straight-line position, the traction can be altered by simply raising or lowering the head of the bed. When the head of the bed is raised, it allows greater pull on the chin and less pull on the occiput. This is necessary in patients who develop severe headaches while being treated in halter traction. Headaches are usually due to overpull of the cervical muscula-

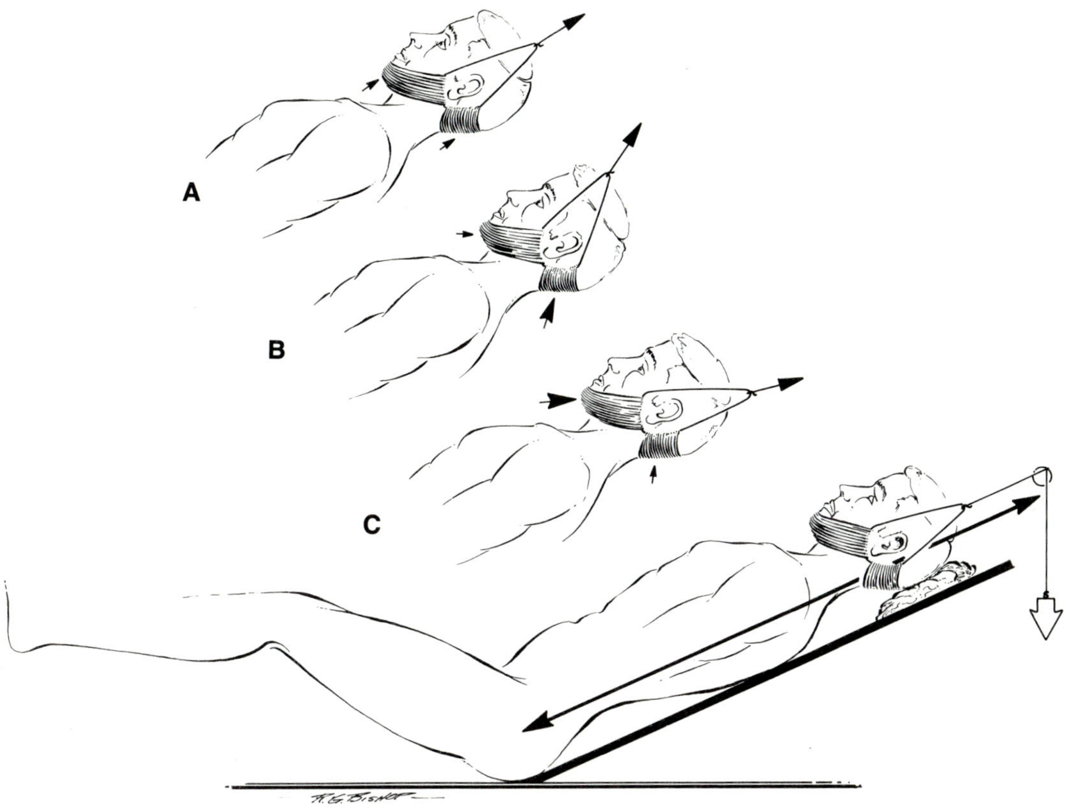

Fig. 2-1. The application of cervical traction in the recumbent position is generally accomplished with the patient in the semiflexed position (*bottom*). With the patient in traction, the head of the bed should be elevated to 30 or 40 degrees, with the hips and knees both flexed approximately 45 degrees. The line of pull should be a straight line from the buttocks to the pulley. Attachment to the head with a cervical halter is shown (*top*). *(A)* When the pull is completely straight, there is equal pressure on the chin and on the occiput. In the event that either of these areas become tender because of continued pull, the pressure may be altered by alterations in the direction of pull. The alteration of pull may be accomplished by leaving the pulley in the same place and raising or lowering the head of the bed, so that the line of pull, in relationship to the long axis of the trunk, is altered. *(B)* If the head of the bed is lowered slightly, the pull is in a more anterior direction, causing less pressure on the chin and more pressure on the occiput. *(C)* If the occiput has become tender and occipital headaches have occurred as a result of the pull, the head of the bed can be raised slightly. This causes the pull to be in a more posterior direction, which causes a greater amount of pressure on the chin and a lesser amount on the occiput.

ture; pain develops at the point of attachment of the cervical musculature to the occiput. Conversely, if the head of the bed is lowered slightly, the ratio of pull becomes greater on the occiput and less on the chin. This is important in patients who develop considerable soreness of the chin, which often occurs with prolonged cervical traction. The pain that occurs in the chin is related to the compression force upon the thin layer of soft tissue that is interposed between the chin portion of the halter and the mandible. Since there is rela-

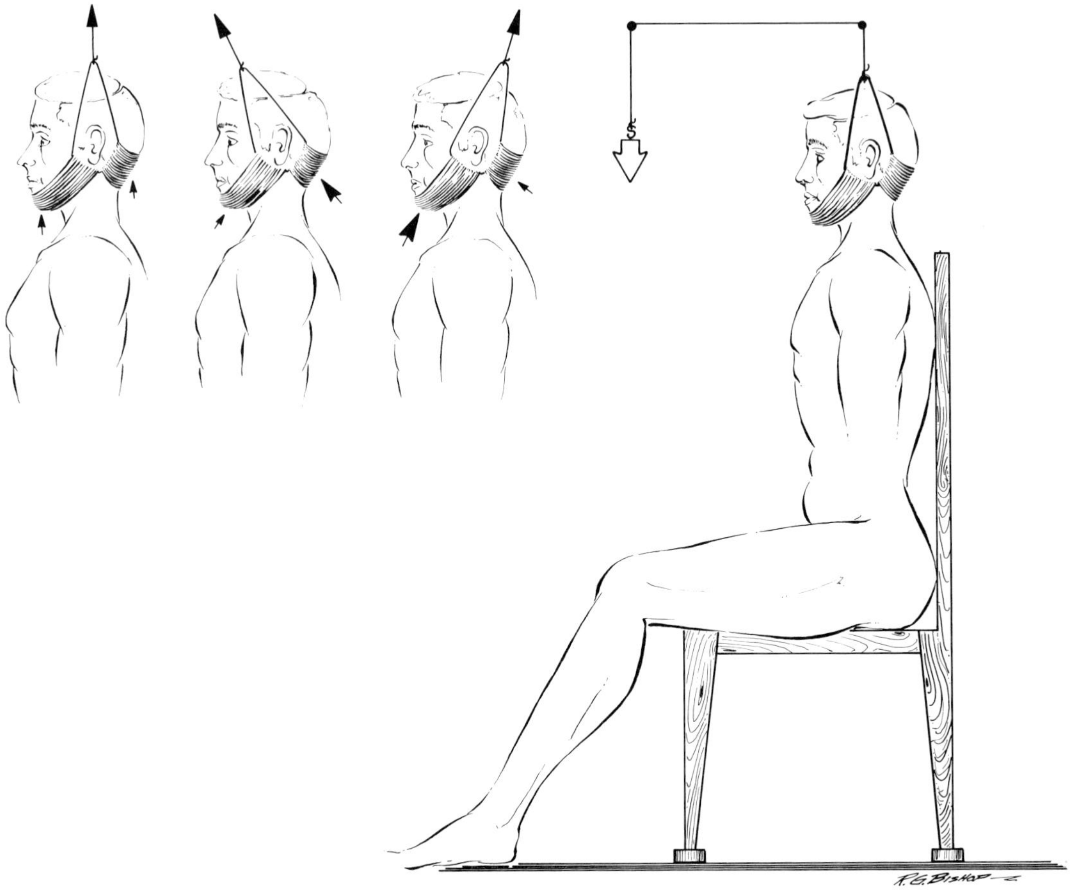

Fig. 2-2. Pull applied with the patient in the erect position is accomplished by using the same type of halter, but with two pulleys that are attached to a doorjamb by eye screws. The traction is applied as shown (*right*), with the amount and duration of traction prescribed by the physician. Ordinarily, 10 minutes of traction with 15 pounds of weight, twice daily, is suitable. The amount of pressure on the occiput or the chin may be varied by moving the chair forward or backward to cause the line of pull to be somewhat more posterior or anterior, respectively.

tively little padding here, this skin is particularly susceptible to pressure; severe pain sometimes results. However, this can be accommodated by the change of position mentioned; the pressure on the chin can be relieved enough to make the traction tolerable for the patient.

Cervical traction by halter is generally applied intermittently. The patient usually can take the traction off himself and periodically get out of bed. Since most of the conditions treated by halter traction are those not involved with stability of the cervical spine, this type of traction does not necessarily need to be extremely efficient. By the same token, it does not need to be continuous, as it does in cases where fractures of the cervical spine exist.

Halter traction also is applied in the sitting position (Fig.2-2). As a matter of fact, the sitting position is probably preferable for the patient who receives traction at home and who does not have the benefit of a hospital bed. Cervical traction in the sitting position is administered usually by a setup which includes two separate pulleys which attach either to the door by a bracket or to the wooden frame of the door. Traction setups are made by various companies for administration of home traction. They generally include not only the halter but also the mechanisms for attachment of the traction apparatus to the door frame. While the amount of traction usually varies, it can be applied in greater amounts, as a general rule, since the period of time in traction is less. Many physicians will order as much as 15 pounds of weight; in the upright position this amount is necessary to overcome the actual weight of the head (7-10 pounds). This amount of weight is usually left on for a period of 10 to 15 minutes, twice daily. For this short period of time, the soft tissue of the chin and the occiput readily tolerate the increased amount of traction. Excessive pressure on the occiput or on the chin may be modified by moving the patient's chair forward or backward enough to cause a shifting of the proportionate pull on the chin or the head, whichever the case may be.

Since the vast majority of the cases that require traction on the cervical spine are those in which instability does not exist, most of the cases requiring cervical traction can be handled very effectively with halter traction. However, when more effective traction is necessary in greater amounts, and when this greater amount of pull must be left on continuously, skeletal attachment to the skull must be used.

Tongs

When instability of the cervical spine exists or when fractures or dislocations occur in the cervical vertebrae, a more efficient type of cervical traction must be administered. Traction that is necessary for these cases must be: (1) traction that is very efficient so that it can be regulated quite closely by the amount of weight applied, (2) traction that can be much greater in amount than that tolerated with the halter, and (3) traction that can be applied continuously 24 hours a day over protracted periods of time. It is necessary in these instances, therefore, to apply skeletal traction. The area of the body that must be attached to the traction is the cranium; an apparatus that will attach to the skull must be utilized. Cranial tongs were described by Crutchfield in 1933 and remain the most popular tongs in use today. (Fig. 2-3*A*). There have been various modifications, such as the Vinke and the Barton tongs, but the basic principle is still that of attachment to the skull. This requires two points of impingement on the lateral aspects of the cranium; pressure between these two areas results in fixation. This allows, then, for pull along the longitudinal line of the cervical spine.

Cranial Halo

The cranial halo described by Perry and Nickel gives a much more efficient skeletal fixation to the skull (Fig. 2-3*C* and *D*). While the halo is more complicated, it allows traction to be applied with better control in the various planes, both lateral and rotatory, so that considerable advantage may be derived from

(Text continued on page 26.)

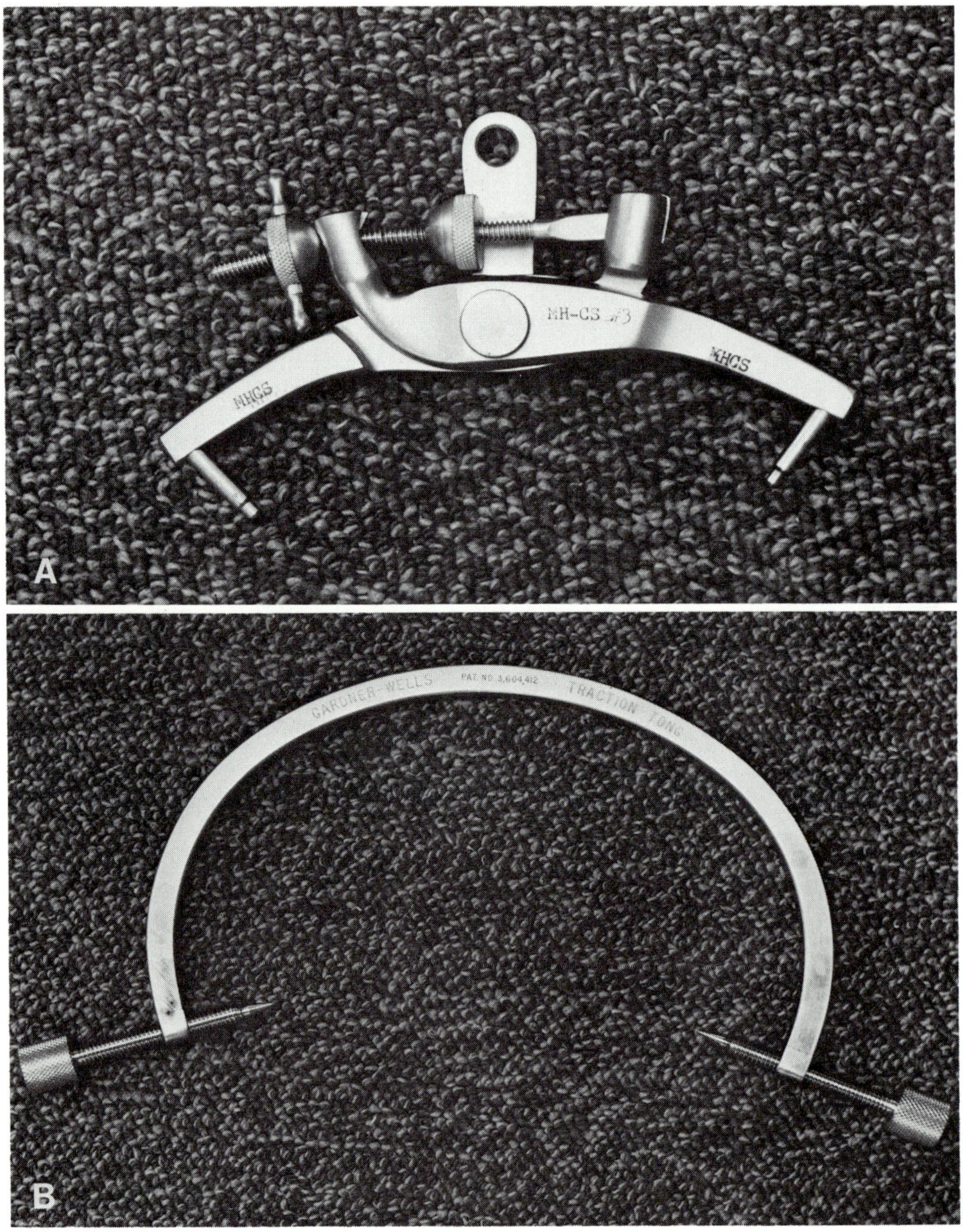

Fig. 2-3. Attachment to the cranium for a more intense and continuous traction may be done by the use of cranial tongs or the cranial halo. *(A and B)* Crutchfield tongs. Note that there is a guard to prevent overpenetration into the skull. Note also that tightening of thumb screw results in tightening of the purchase of the skull. Traction is produced by pull on the opposite end of the tongs. It can be altered by attachment farther to one side than the other. (*Legend continued on opposite page.*)

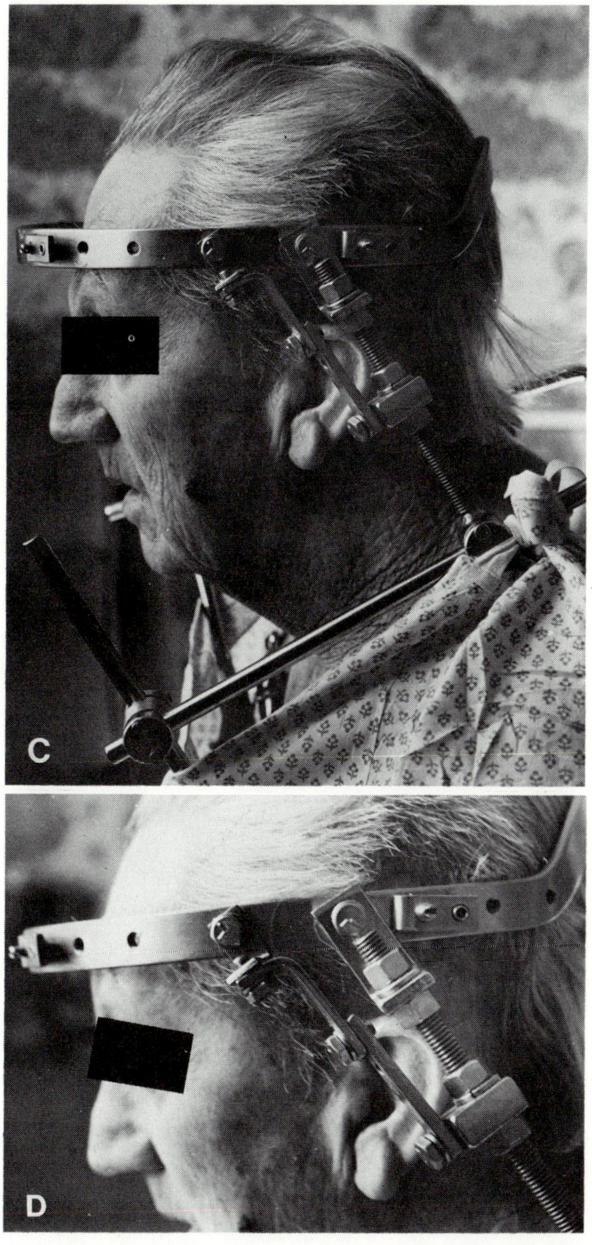

Fig. 2-3, continued. (C and D) Cranial halo. The halo is attached to the skull by pins that impinge upon the skull at the four quadrants. Attachment is shown to the body component, which has been incorporated to a plaster-of-paris cast. Variations in position can be achieved by alterations in the device that attaches the halo to the supporting structures.

this traction. It is also possible to provide ambulatory traction using the cranial halo. After the fracture has been reduced and stabilized with the patient in the supine position, the halo may be fixed to an outrigger suspended above a plaster body jacket.

Crutchfield tongs can be applied under a local anesthetic in the emergency room, and the appropriate traction can be applied. These tongs have a guard to prevent overpenetration through the skull. However, they have a tendency to loosen somewhat, due to pressure necrosis of the bone; it is necessary to tighten them at least daily. By the same token, the halo attachment to the skull depends upon four separate pins which impinge into the skull at the four quadrants of the circumference of the skull. It is necessary for these pins to be tightened with a 5-pound torque screwdriver. This should be done daily so that they will stay well impinged upon the skull.

The amount of traction that can be applied through Crutchfield tongs or the halo apparatus varies according to the condition being treated. As a general rule, 10 pounds of weight is required to overcome the weight of the head as it impinges against the underlying mattress or sling. In addition, traction must be applied to stabilize the fracture or reduce the fracture dislocation. It is seldom necessary to apply more than 40 pounds of weight to the device. Reduction that does not occur over a period of 24 hours with this amount of weight most likely represents an irreducible fracture that will require surgical reduction. Position can be altered slightly, particularly in rotation, if it appears that this will help secure reduction of dislocations of the cervical spine facets. Very frequent x-ray examinations should be done with the portable machine to monitor the position of the vertebrae and the overall effect of traction.

Special Beds

Onc of the basic problems that exists when skeletal traction is being applied to the cervical spine is that the patient must lie immobile for long periods of time. This results in pressure phenomena to the portion of the body touching the bed or frame. It is for this reason that a special apparatus must be used, which can allow for turning without changing the line of pull or the effectiveness of the traction.

The Stryker or "sandwich" bed has gained wide popularity; it probably constitutes the best method of caring for individuals who must lie motionless in the horizontal position for long periods of time (Fig. 2-4*A* and *B*). The apparatus consists of two separate frames with canvas bottoms, which are joined with the patient sandwiched between them. Once the sandwich has been created with the frames on either side of the patient, a latch is released which allows the entire apparatus to rotate one-half turn, so that the patient, previously lying on his back, is turned to his abdomen without actually moving his body. The mechanism of this bed is quite simple. The patient lying on his back on Frame A has but to have Frame B applied over his anterior side and straps applied to hold the two frames closely together, with the patient interposed. When the latch is released and the frame is turned over, the top frame can be removed leaving the patient lying on his anterior side with his posterior side completely exposed. The patients in this apparatus generally are turned frequently, usually at 4- to 6-hour intervals. In this way, care can be given to the skin and pressure areas.

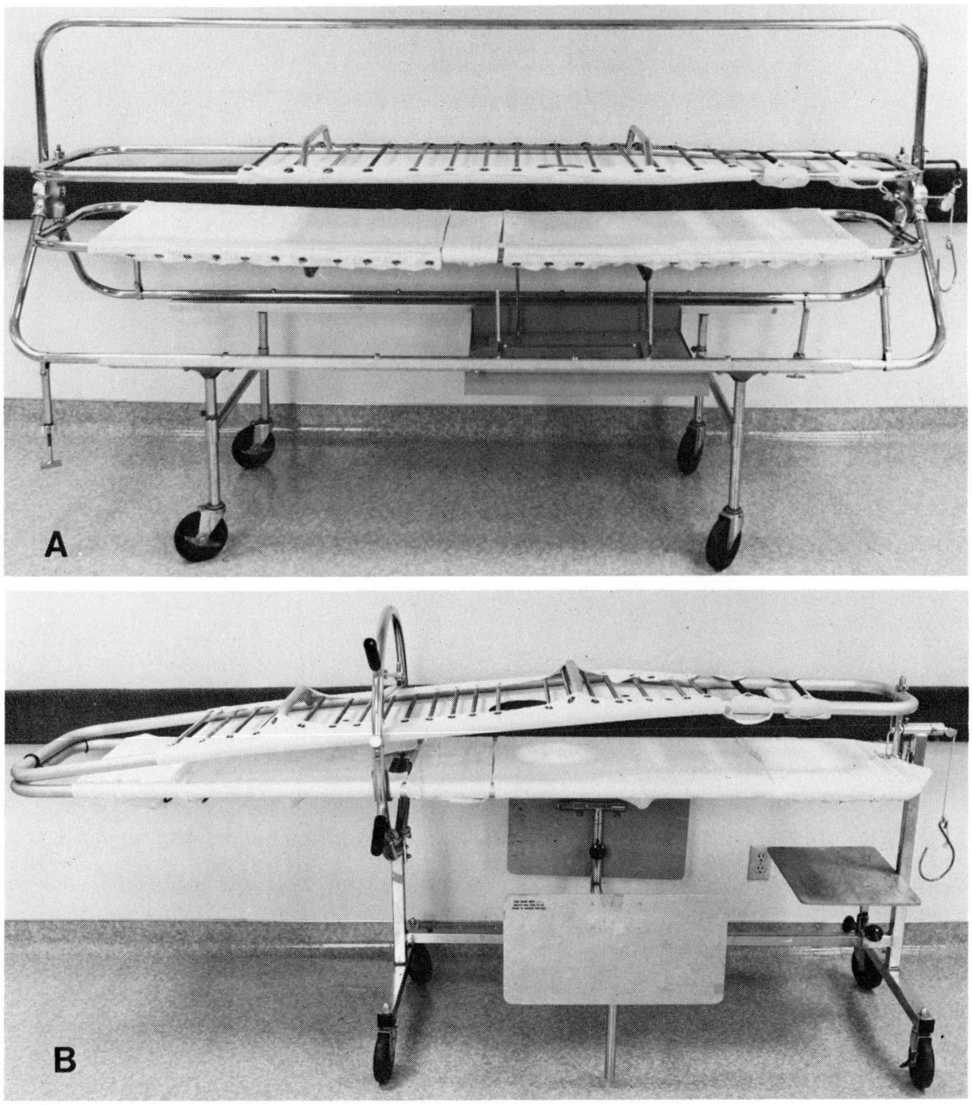

Fig. 2-4. For a patient in cervical traction with cranial tongs where motion through the cervical spine is to be avoided, the use of a special apparatus is necessary for turning the patient. *(A and B)* Two models of a Stryker frame or "sandwich bed." The patient is placed on one half of the bed, either on his back or prone. To turn him, the opposite side of the frame is applied to the exposed side and fastened securely, so that the patient is encased between the two halves, much as in a sandwich position. The entire frame is turned on its pivots on either end, so that the patient is completely turned over onto his opposite side. The superior half of the frame is then removed. When this procedure has been completed, the patient has been satisfactorily turned without actually having moved his body. *(Continued on next page.)*

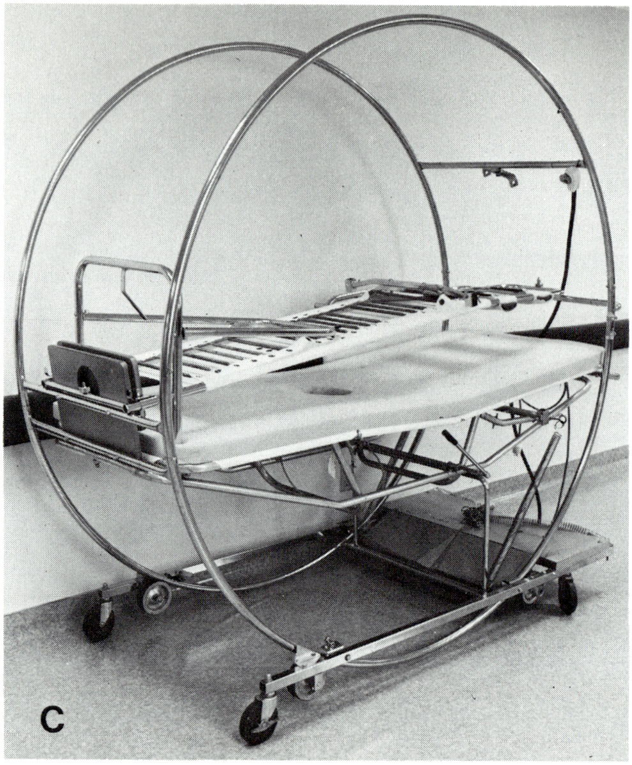

Fig. 2-4, continued. (C) The CircOlectric bed. This bed accomplishes a similar function, except that the patient is turned in an end-over-end direction, rather than in a side-to-side direction. A restraining frame is placed over the exposed side. Once the bed has been turned 180 degrees, the opposite side is removed. The CircOlectric bed is much more expensive, but it can be stopped in any position. The patient can be turned gradually or can be tilted in any desired position by stopping the mechanism at any point.

Ordinarily, when greater amounts of weight are used in cervical traction, a heavy wire is used instead of rope to attach the weights through a pulley to the skeletal fixation device, whether tongs or halo. The wire passes through a tiny opening at the end of the frame, so that the longitudinal traction is continued during the turning process. No matter whether the patient lies on his ventral or dorsal side, the traction continues uninterrupted.

CircOlectric Bed. This is a more recent modification of the Stryker frame. This bed provides the same convenience in turning, but allows for the turning in an end-over-end direction, rather than in a lateral direction (Fig. 2-4*C*). The patient's body lies horizontally in the circular frame, and constitutes the horizontal diameter of the circle. The same sandwich mechanism is used as with the Stryker, but the electrical system in the bed rotates the circle. The patient passes head over feet to change from the ventral to the dorsal position. The CircOlectric bed is much more expensive and much more cumbersome; its use has not gained the widespread popularity that is enjoyed by the Stryker frame. This CircOlectric bed does have the advantage that it can be stopped in various positions; the patient can be tilted slightly head-up or head-down, while still retaining the horizontal position and still maintaining longitudinal traction.

UPPER EXTREMITY

Traction on the upper extremity is usually necessary for fractures or injuries involving the shoulder, the shoulder girdle, or the humerus. Elbow fractures require traction for maintenance of position, and occasionally the traction is applied in such a manner that the arm is suspended over the anterior aspect of the body, so that venous drainage is improved and swelling diminished. The same fundamental principles apply to upper extremity traction. Fixation to the extremity is provided either by a pin through the bone, or by straps attached to the skin. An additional type of traction that is used in fractures involving the humerus or elbow is the so-called Dunlops traction (Fig. 2-5). A soft sling is used to pull against the forearm, which is flexed at slightly greater than 90 degrees with the upper arm. The hand and the forearm are suspended in a balanced traction to keep the sling in place.

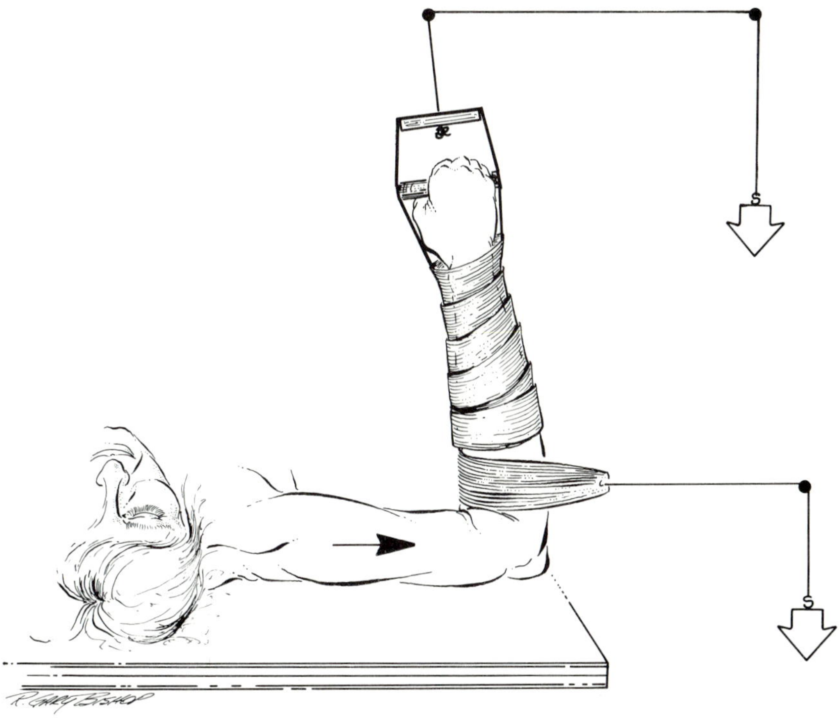

Fig. 2-5. Dunlop's traction. This setup is for longitudinal traction on the humerus when only temporary traction is desired and when the amount of weight necessary is not great. The arm must be bent at slightly more than 90 degrees. A suspension apparatus is applied to the forearm with traction straps and an elastic wrap, utilizing only enough weight to hold the forearm upright and the elbow just touching the bed. The pulley above the hand is placed slightly toward the shoulder, so that the elbow can be flexed at slightly more than 90 degrees. The sling at the proximal forearm must be well padded and fashioned in such a manner that the margin does not create a ridge at the bend of the elbow. A moderate amount of traction, up to 5 or 6 pounds, can be applied for rather extended periods of time, provided that the condition of the soft tissue underneath the sling is inspected periodically. If more weight is necessary, or if a protracted time in traction is anticipated, consideration should be given to skeletal traction by a pin drilled through the olecranon.

Side-arm Traction

When traction is to be applied to the upper extremity, the extremity is usually moved out from the body and suspended in a frame to constitute a balanced traction. If traction is necessary for some length of time, particularly when the fracture exists in the distal humerus or elbow, pin traction through the olecranon is desirable. It is much more efficient and allows for fixation to the extremity without circumferential wrappings.

A good example of the necessity for skeletal traction is shown in the supracondylar fracture of the elbow, especially when swelling is great enough to preclude putting the elbow in the flexion necessary to maintain position of the distal fragment (Fig. 2-6). In those instances when swelling is great enough to impede circulation, the elbow is placed in less than 90 degrees of flexion. A pin is drilled through the olecranon. Satisfactory longitudinal traction can be applied to the humerus. Flexion of the distal fragment, in relationship to the shaft fragment, is possible without the necessity of flexing the elbow joint,

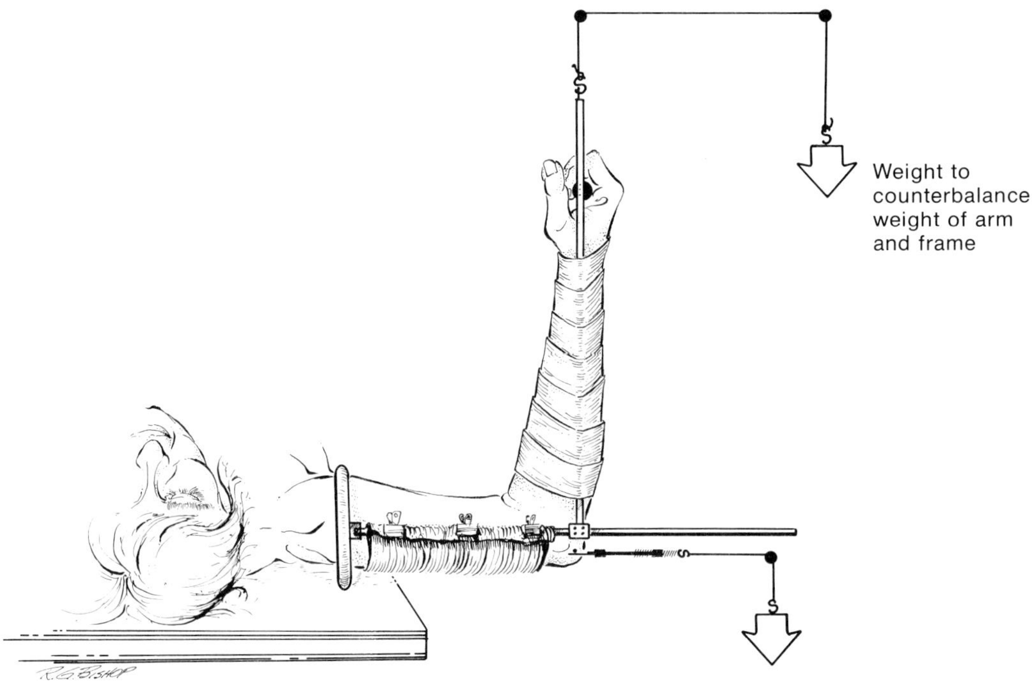

Fig. 2-6. Balanced side-arm traction. The arm is passed through the ring, which is then passed up so that it encompasses the shoulder. The upright attachment for the forearm may be moved in either direction to accommodate the length of the humerus. A cloth sling is placed on the horizontal segment to provide a surface on which the arm may rest. The olecranon extends just past the vertical limb, so that the pin drilled through the olecranon will be clear and allow unimpeded traction. The forearm is placed between the two upright supports, and usually held there with a circumferentially applied elastic bandage. A rope is attached to the vertical section and is passed through pulleys. A weight is attached to exactly counterbalance the weight of the arm and the frame. Skeletal traction is then applied in the desired amount through the pin in the olecranon. The entire extremity is counterbalanced so that a balanced traction system is created.

itself. This traction also lends itself to an "over the face" traction which also greatly reduces swelling by creating a very effective elevation of the extremity (Fig. 2-7). Comminuted fractures of the humerus are likewise often treated, in the initial stages, by balanced side-arm traction until the fragments become fused enough to allow ambulation in a hanging cast, as described below. In all of these instances, the countertraction is accomplished by the weight of the body.

Forearm Traction

While forearm traction is not often indicated, there may be instances when fractures of the distal radius and ulna are treated with traction to allow for improvement of the circulation before further definitive treatment is done. It is virtually impossible to apply traction to the forearm with other than skeletal fixation; the forearm does not lend itself to skin attachments.

When skeletal fixation is necessary, it is accomplished by drilling a small-size Kirschner wire transversely across and through the shaft of the third and fourth metacarpals, attaching it to a traction bow. This gives good, stable fixation to the bone and allows for pull along the longitudinal axis of the forearm. It is necessary to stabilize the upper arm and elbow for countertraction. This can be done with traction tapes to apply longitudinal traction to the humerus for support. It can also be done by placing a sandbag across the arm to act as countertraction.

Portable Traction

The upper extremity lends itself to portable traction more readily than most any other type of traction; the patient can be ambulatory and still maintain the traction device.

Hanging Casts. A good example is the hanging cast applied for ambulatory traction in the longitudinal axis of the humerus (Fig. 2-8). The cast acts only as a weight and has nothing to do with stability of the fracture, from a coaptation standpoint. It often is found that fractures of the upper humerus are treated with a hanging cast that does not even come up to the level of the fracture. It is important to explain these concepts to the patient so that he understands the objective in mind, and will not be dismayed when he finds that the cast does not cover the fracture site.

There are several important points about hanging casts that should be mentioned. It is necessary for the cast to be applied with the elbow at more than 90 degrees of flexion. The fact that the elbow is acutely flexed allows for the weight to be applied strictly to the long axis of the humerus without any deforming angulatory factors.

It is necessary for the suspension to occur at a point opposite the radial styloid, so that the mechanical fulcrum can be established there; the lever arm applies longitudinal traction in the long axis of the humerus. The point of attachment of the single band supporting the cast should be at the radial styloid. If it is in this position, with the elbow flexed at more than 90 degrees, the lever arm will act mechanically to provide the longitudinal traction.

Probably the most important consideration is that the patient stays in the upright position at all times, even while asleep. The hospital bed should have the back elevated to maximal height, or the bed at home should have the back

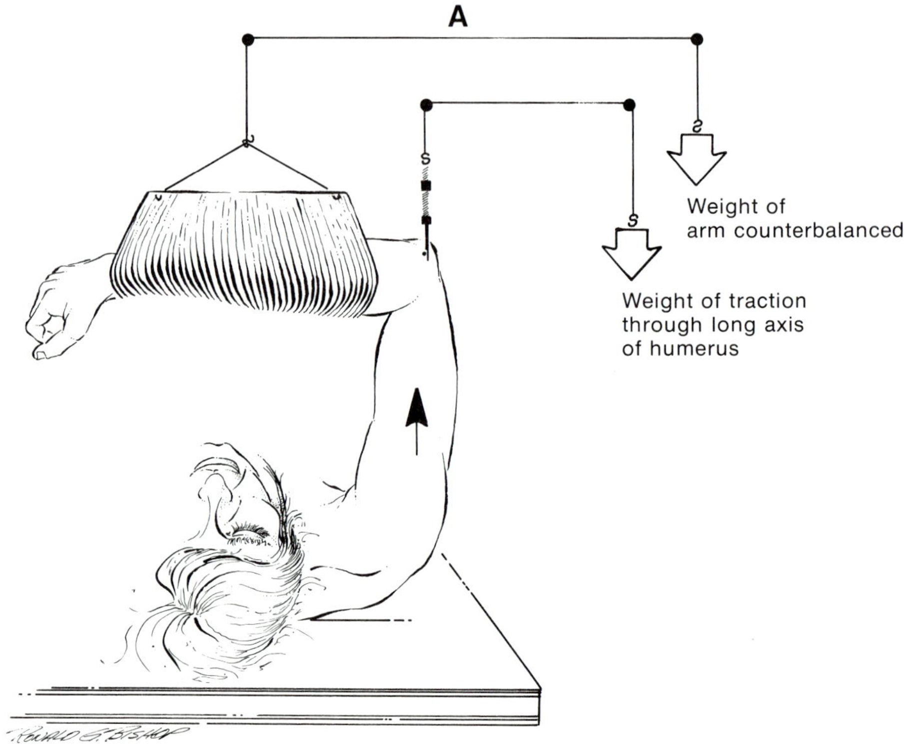
A
Weight of
arm counterbalanced
Weight of traction
through long axis
of humerus

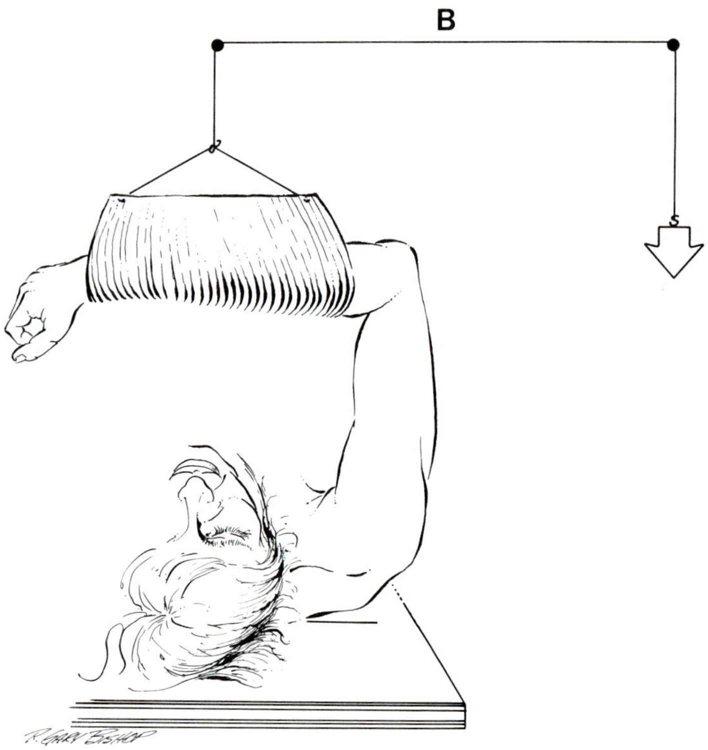
B

elevated to insure effectiveness of the traction during sleeping hours. When the patient lies down no traction exists, and the hanging cast is entirely useless.

Another word of caution concerns the weight of the cast. Probably the most important complication of treating fractures with a hanging cast is nonunion with distraction of the fracture ends if the cast is too heavy. There is a tendency to feel that the cast must be quite heavy to accomplish the desired result, but minimal weight is usually all that is necessary to reduce and maintain position of humeral shaft fractures. Therefore, the cast should not be heavy at all. Again, serial roentgenograms should be taken to ascertain the position of the fracture to determine whether additional traction should be added, or whether some of the traction should be removed by cutting off a portion of the cast with the electric cast saw.

A final word of caution concerns using this traction apparatus with obese patients or with female patients with unusually large breasts. In the obese patient, it is difficult to maintain the longitudinal position of the humerus. The chest wall will create an angular deforming feature; external bowing of the fracture often results. This is even more true in women with pendulous breasts that impinge upon the side of the cast and produce lateral angulation at the fracture site. Slight correction may be possible by changing the attachment ring's relation to the radial styloid. By placing the ring slightly more volarward (but still at the styloid level), the forearm is rotated slightly, helping to correct angulation of the humerus toward the body. The converse is true when the ring is placed slightly dorsalward and the pressure is placed on the humerus to correct outward bowing. This is shown in Figure 2-8.

If all these factors are carefully observed, hanging casts are an excellent method of ambulatory treatment of humeral shaft fractures and fractures about the humeral head and shoulder. Careful monitoring by roentgenogram is mandatory to be certain that the fracture is held in the desirable position, and that deforming factors do not develop. As mentioned earlier, it often is better also to apply side-arm balanced traction for a period of time, early in the course of treatment. This maintains the fracture in the desired position while the fragments become adherent to one another; when the hanging cast is applied, there is little chance for disengagement of the fragments.

Hand Fractures. Portable traction also is used occasionally in hand fractures. The old banjo splint, in which the circular outrigger traction apparatus was applied over the tips of the extended fingers, is mentioned only to condemn it.

←

Fig. 2-7. (Opposite) (A) Occasionally, longitudinal traction can be placed in the long axis of the humerus with the arm suspended over the face. The pin through the olecranon again serves as the fixation to the extremity. The placement of the humerus with relationship to the traction allows for longitudinal pull and negation of the effect of gravity, as described in Figure 1-4 for the lower extremity. The forearm is then supported in a second pulley setup by means of a cloth sling. The weight must be just sufficient to counterbalance the weight of the forearm. This type of traction adheres to the principles of balanced traction, but does not require the carrier for the extremity. It also allows for better elevation of the part, to prevent swelling. *(B)* The suspension of an extremity without pin traction. This setup is used in instances where elevation is necessary for the prevention or treatment of swelling of the forearm, hand, or elbow.

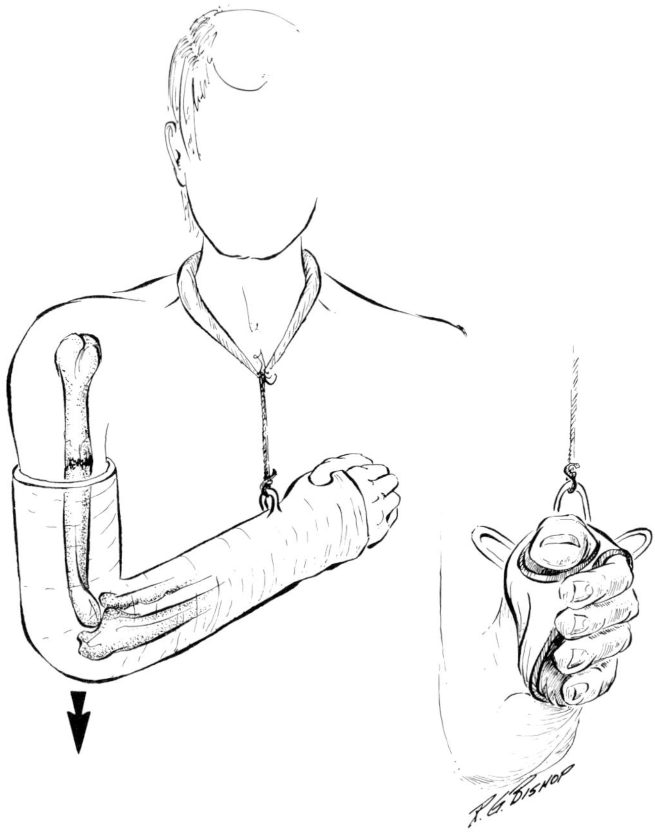

Fig. 2-8. Hanging-cast traction for the humerus or shoulder. The cast must be precisely applied to be effective. The cast does not necessarily need to come above the fracture site *per se*, since it supplies weight and traction rather than immobilization. It may be of some additional stability to apply the cast up over the fracture site, if this is feasible. The elbow must be flexed more than 90 degrees. The only point of attachment is by means of a loop placed at the radial styloid. A ring is formed of plaster, as the cast is being applied, for attachment of the sling. The sling need be only a padded collar with a length of cord or rope attached for attachment to the styloid ring. some control of rotation can be accomplished by variation in the location of the styloid ring (*inset*). The rings on the dorsal or palmar side allow for some correction of angulation at the fracture site. The weight of the cast gives longitudinal traction through the long axis of the humerus only when the erect position is maintained. The cast is ineffective when the patient is lying down. The cast is likewise ineffective when the patient supports it on a pillow or when a sling other than the suspension cord is used.

Any traction applied to the fingers must be with the proximal joints in flexion to preclude contractures in the collateral ligaments, resulting in permanent loss of extension. Bunnell pointed out many years ago that the collateral ligaments of the proximal joints are in their longest position with the joint in 90 degrees of flexion. If the joint is held in complete extension for any period of time, the collateral ligaments contract and become shortened. Flexion is no longer possible without surgical release of the contracted ligaments. It is therefore mandatory that any traction applied to the hand be with the fingers in the flexed position.

Attachment to the fingers usually is accomplished with a small Kirschner wire through the distal phalanx. Occasionally, adhesive tape straps are used to hold the finger to the rubberband, which is the motor power for the traction. The amount of traction necessary to immobilize or reduce fractures of the fingers is very small; care must be taken to avoid overpull. The reader is referred to standard textbooks concerning the treatment of hand fractures.

LOWER EXTREMITY

The use of traction probably is more appropriate in conditions involving the lower extremity than it is in most other regions of the body. It will be recalled that much of the discussion concerning the application of traction utilized the lower extremity for examples. Whereas there are relatively few indications for balanced traction in the upper extremity, traction in the lower extremity is a time-honored practice.

Along with its use for fractures of the lower extremity, traction on the leg is also used as an adjunct to treatment of other conditions. Traction on a single leg is useful in immobilizing the extremity following a closed reduction of a dislocated hip. The leg is kept in traction for 3 weeks to allow for capsular healing. This is ususally a skin traction setup, but nevertheless, it is traction on the lower extremity. Many fractures of the pelvis necessitate the application of traction to either one or both of the lower extremities. With the advent of newer methods for internal fixation, traction for treatment of fractures of the femur became less commonly used. Internal fixation allows for earlier mobilization, which cuts down on hospital stay, and prevents many conditions related to long continuous bedrest. There still are some instances, however, in which badly comminuted fractures of the femur are treated by traction alone when an open reduction is not feasible. There still are many femoral fractures that are treated by balanced traction in the hospital.

Traction on the lower extremity is the treatment of choice in fractures of the femur in children. Open reduction is seldom indicated; practically all femoral fractures in prepubertal patients are treated with traction. Since the mechanism of traction varies considerably with different indications, it is necessary to discuss separately each of the types of lower-extremity traction.

Buck's Traction

The simplest and most commonly used longitudinal traction in the lower extremity is Buck's traction. This is a simple straight-leg traction that is not of the balanced variety. It may be applied to one or both legs simultaneously. It is not a particularly effective traction; it does not exert a tremendous amount of pull on the extremity. It is not effective particularly since the extremity lies on the bed; the pull merely exerts a certain amount of longitudinal force along the long axis of the extremity, especially from the knee down. More often, this traction is used as a holding mechanism; the extremity can be immobilized with a moderate amount of pull. As mentioned previously, it is not possible to apply a great amount of traction with skin attachments. It is seldom possible to apply more than 5 or 6 pounds of Buck's traction, especially if the pull is to be exerted over any length of time. This traction is used to stabilize the extremity, and often is used for injuries to the hip or leg that are not severe enough to require the more exacting skeletal traction. As an example, a dislocated hip that has been reduced by closed manipulation is usually held with a simple Buck's traction; the traction affords both immobilization and a moderate amount of pull on the extremity to relax muscle spasm.

Low Back Pain. Much of the time, Buck's traction is applied for low back pain with nerve root irritation and pain extending down into the extremity. While many operators now much prefer pelvic traction rather than single extremity traction, the latter is still occasionally used. When Buck's traction *is* applied in the treatment of low back pain, it is necessary that it be applied with the hip and the knee flexed, as shown in Figure 2-9. It is only with the patient in this position that the hamstring muscles and the sciatic nerve are relaxed, so that pain is not aggravated by the position alone. It is quite easy, particularly if the hip is flexed with the knee straight, to apply considerable stretch on the sciatic nerve with this traction, aggravating the condition being treated.

Fractures of the Hip. Buck's traction also is often utilized for the interim treatment of fractures of the hip while the patient is awaiting more definitive surgical fixation. The traction is applied basically as a matter of comfort and, again, to immobilize the extremity and prevent further damage at the fracture site. Even though the leg is held fairly straight, a rolled towel or sheet can be placed under the knee to give the small amount of flexion necessary to secure more comfort.

Attachment. Buck's traction is applied with attachment to the extremity by means of either skin tapes or a foam rubber padded boot.

When skin strips are used, they usually are fashioned from adhesive strips or mole skin, which adheres to the lateral aspects of the leg, and is secured with an elastic wrap over the straps. Care must be taken to pad the malleoli carefully, with the spreader bar or block at the end of the tapes being wide enough to preclude undue pressure across the malleoli. The spreader block is attached to a single rope, which is stretched in a longitudinal fashion along the long axis of the extremity, passed through a single pulley, and attached to the appropriate amount of weight. Skin attachment has the disadvantage of requiring adhesion to the skin, and many times blistering will occur. An alternative skin fixation can be foam rubber padded straps applied to the extremity—the foam rubber facing the skin—and the external circumference wrapped with elastic bandages tightly enough so that the sponge rubber does not slip on the skin. This requires relatively new tapes; any grease that forms on the skin will

Fig. 2-9. (Opposite) (A) Buck's traction application should be in the position shown *(bottom)*, with the hips and knees flexed, and the patient should be kept preferably in a hospital-type bed. Attachment to the extremity may be either by straps *(top)* or by the polyfoam boot. *(B and C)* A unique type of polyfoam boot is marketed under the trade name of Medsco. The traction straps are attached to the sole portion of the boot. They then pass through rings on either side, so that as traction is applied to the entire boot, there occurs a compression under the sole of the foot. This permits a better fit and prevents the tendency of the foot to drop into equinus as the traction is applied. This boot is felt to be superior to other types that do not have this feature.

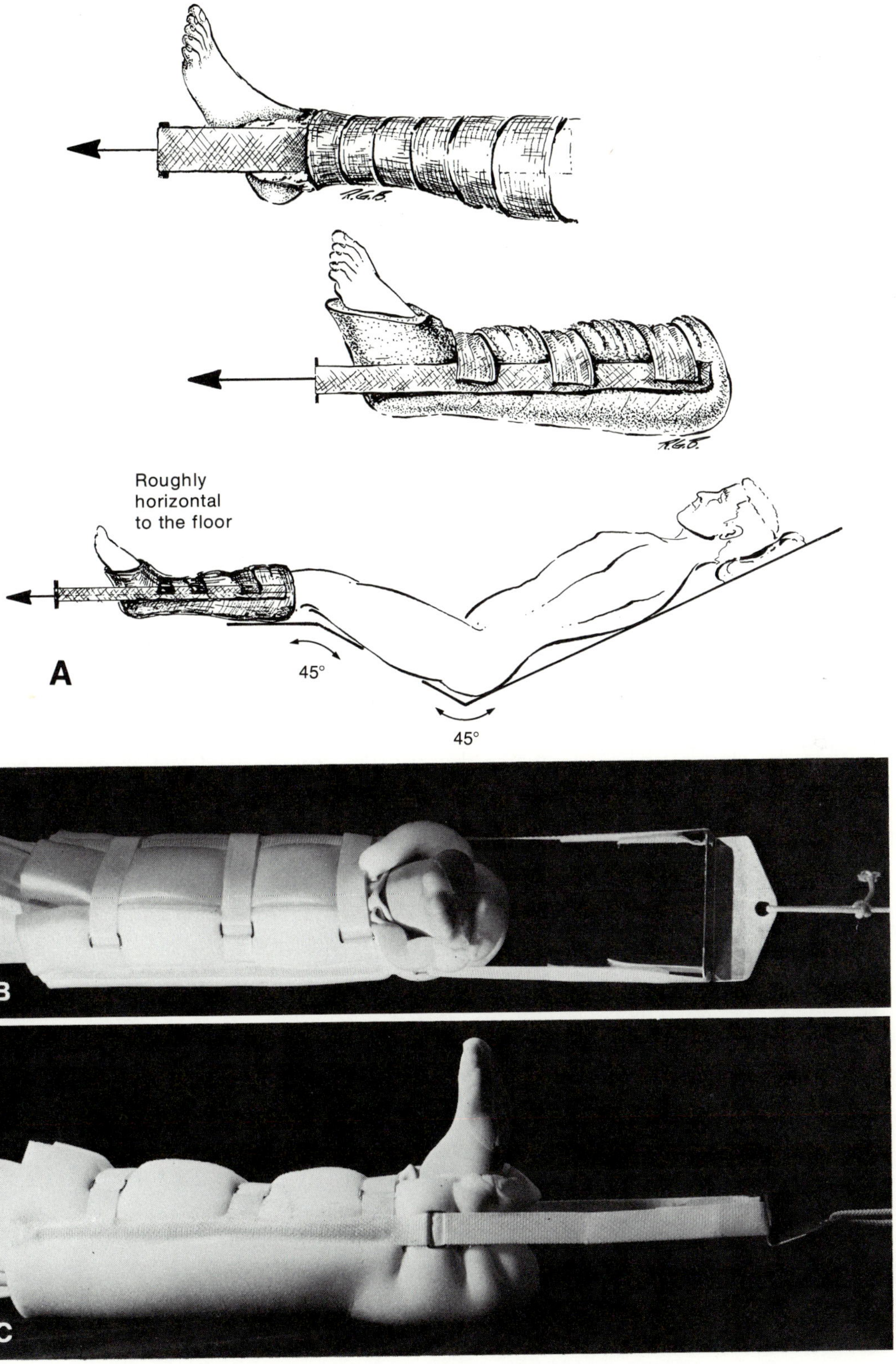
Roughly
horizontal
to the floor
A
45°
45°
B
C

ultimately increase the chances of slipping and cause the traction to become ineffective. A word of caution here concerns the use of circumferential wrapping. It must be loose enough to prevent impairment of the circulation, but it should be tight enough to afford good contact between the sponge rubber tapes and the skin. The circumferential wrappings should be reapplied at least once daily, and perhaps every 12 hours, to prevent any damage to the skin. These straps are relatively thin, the layer of sponge rubber being relatively small. Most manufacturers supply them with multiple tiny perforations in the sponge rubber, so that perspiration is not allowed to accumulate and maceration of the skin is less likely to occur.

Foam Rubber Boot. More recently, the foam rubber boot has become popular as a method of attaching traction to the skin. It seems to fulfill most of the necessities of traction, while obviating many of the disadvantages. The boots are made of thick polyfoam which is soft and pliable enough to afford a good cushioning effect to the skin. The boot is applied, as shown in Figure 2-9 (center), with straps holding the open side of the boot together tightly enough to afford traction at the point of contact of the polyfoam to the skin. The disadvantage of some boots is that they tend to slip down slightly and the foot falls into equinus. This is a disadvantage of the other types of Buck's traction attachments when tapes are used and when no counterpressure is placed against the foot. A boot has been manufactured by Medical Specialties Company,* which has a mechanism whereby the traction is applied through tapes which originate at the distal end of the boot. They pass through rings on either side, so that the longitudinal traction also forces the bottom of the boot up against the plantar surface of the foot. This gives a much better contact, is much more comfortable, and prevents the foot from falling into equinus while traction is being applied. These boots should be loosened several times daily so that the skin may be allowed to dry and the condition of the skin may be observed. Since this boot does apply rather even pressure over the entire lower part of the extremity with only the distal portion of the forefoot being exposed, there is much less chance for swelling, circumferential banding, and other sources of circulatory interference to occur.

Bryant's Traction

Bryant's traction is utilized in children, usually in treatment of fractures of the femur. This traction is not used in youngsters that weigh more than 40 pounds (18 kg.). The reason for the weight limitation is that Bryant's traction has several real disadvantages when used in heavier youngsters. Severe complications may occur when it is not properly used.

The traction is ordinarily applied to both extremities, even though only one is being actively treated. By applying it to both extremities, the youngster is more appropriately immobilized and the countertraction which is provided by the body is more easily controlled. The amount of weight used is that necessary to apply enough traction so that the buttocks just clear the bed. The amount of weight should not be excessive so that the buttocks are pulled completely off the mattress. It should be regulated so that the skin just touches the mattress when both legs are suspended (Fig. 2-10). Care must be taken to

*Lubbock, Texas.

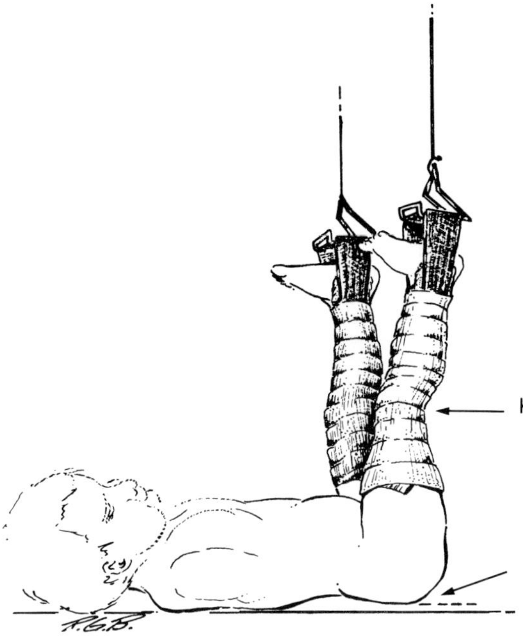

Fig. 2-10. Bryant's traction, for use in femoral fractures in children under 40 pounds (18 kilograms). Traction is usually applied to both legs by traction straps that extend the entire length of the extremity. Several points of caution are necessary: (1) The knee should not be hyperextended. The pulley directly over the feet should lie slightly distal to the buttocks so that the leg, instead of being in a straight perpendicular position, is tilted slightly toward the foot of the bed. This prevents the tendency to hyperextend the knee. (2) The weight applied should be just sufficient to hold the child suspended, so that the buttocks barely touch the bed. (3) The circulation should be closely watched, particularly in older and heavier children.

prevent hyperextension at the knee, the basic cause of difficulty in these patients. When the traction is applied with the overhead pulley too far cephalad, the knee is hyperextended. The vessels are stretched at the knee, and circulatory embarrassment occurs. The overhead pulley should be placed just slightly caudal to the pelvis so that the position of the leg is not hyperextension of the knee. Another real danger is that too much tightness in the circumferential wrappings will result in diminution of circulation.

The position achieved by Bryant's traction (the legs point straight up over the body), provides a considerable strain on the circulation to the feet, due to the hydrostatic pressure against the vascular column. Blood is pumped against gravity to reach the foot. Any additional impediment to the flow of blood renders the circulation inadequate, and circulatory changes may occur. They are more likely to occur with the knee in hyperextension and in the youngster who weighs more than the prescribed 40 pounds; since the amount of traction is greater, the stretching of his leg is likely to be more profound. Similarly, larger youngsters tend to have tighter hamstring muscles which likewise cause increased pressure on the circulation. The circulatory complications are of great magnitude. When they do occur, they occur gradually. Very frequent monitoring of the circulation in the feet should be done, particularly during the first few days following application of traction. Vascular impairment to the extremity is also likely to cause severe pain. Youngsters who are having pain that seems out of proportion to what one would expect in their injury should be suspected of having circulatory impairment in the structures distal to the knee. If any question arises as to the adequacy of circulation, Bryant's traction should be discontinued. A longitudinal traction with pin fixation to the femur should be substituted. In no instance should Bryant's traction be continued when there is questionable circulation distal to the knee.

Once Bryant's traction has been appropriately applied in the appropriate-sized youngster, it will be found that a very comfortable traction exists. Before many days pass, the youngster will move about with great freedom, even though both extremities are suspended in the traction. It is surprising what contortions these youngsters can get into, once the pain has subsided and some healing has occurred at the fracture site. The traction is maintained until the fracture is solid enough that a spica cast can be applied for transportation of the youngster to his home. This can be determined only by serial roentgenograms; they should be done not only to ascertain the amount of healing but also to be certain that adequate reduction of the fracture has occurred. In an occasional instance in which anterior angulation at the fracture site occurs, and when it cannot be corrected with traction over a period of several days, the uninvolved extremity can be removed from the traction. This procedure applies enough rotatory force on the pelvis that sometimes the anterior bow can be corrected. It does not seem to jeopardize the effectiveness of the traction but, as mentioned earlier, it does make the patient harder to control with one extremity that can be moved about at will. When Bryant's traction is applied unilaterally, it is important to monitor the effectiveness of the traction on the involved extremity even more closely, since control is more difficult to achieve.

Balanced Traction For Femoral Or Pelvic Fractures

Perhaps the most classical of all tractions is a balanced traction setup used for treatment of a fracture of the femur. This traction incorporates all of the basic principles of traction application, and it represents the time-honored method of treating this fracture. Much of the earlier discussion in this book concerning the various principles of traction has utilized the concept of a balanced traction apparatus for treatment of lower extremity fractures. A balanced traction setup creates a single unit from the entire extremity; any motion occurs at the hip joint rather than at the fracture site. The balanced traction comprises the most comfortable traction, particularly when it is necessary for long periods of time. If the frame can be adjusted to the point where it is completely comfortable, and if it is perfectly counterbalanced so that the extremity may be raised or lowered voluntarily without difficulty, and when the frame stays in the new location, the traction is quite comfortable and effective.

Attachment. While it is usually the case that balanced traction for femoral or pelvic fractures utilizes pin attachment to the extremity, and skeletal traction, rather than boot or strap traction, it is possible to use the latter. This is done for short periods of time. An example might be the fracture of the femur. The femur is held temporarily in a balanced traction setup, with either boot or strap

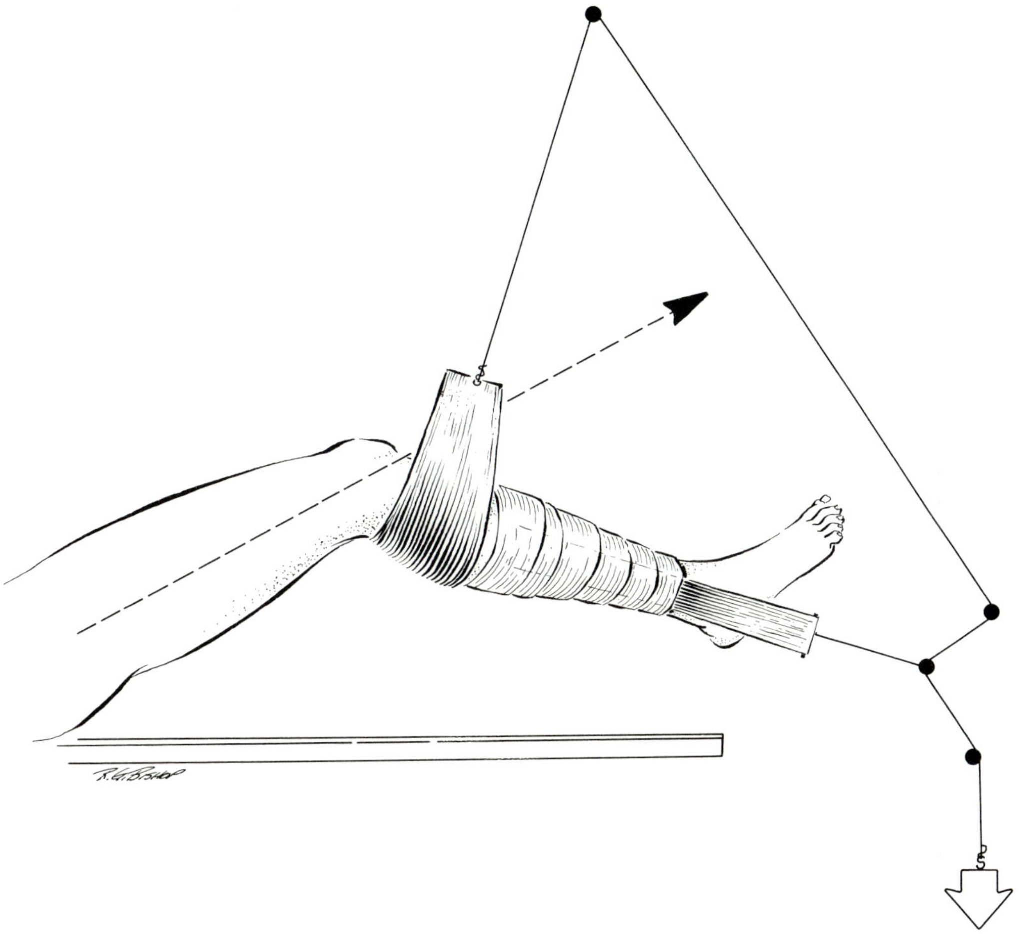

Fig. 2-11. In Russell's double traction, a single weight is used for the suspension of the leg as well as for the longitudinal traction. Note that the sling pulls up on the leg at approximately 45 degrees to the long axis of the femur, while they traction strips on the lower leg pull slightly downward, again, at approximately 45 degrees of pull to the long axis of the femur. This results in a vectored line of pull which is roughly along the long axis of the femur. As might be expected, this type of traction requires frequent adjustment and the frequent taking of roentgenograms to be certain that the traction is adequate.

attachment to the lower extremity, until the patient's general condition improves enough to warrant going ahead with the regular traction setup, or perhaps with open reduction and discontinuation of traction. The simple strap or boot traction does allow for a certain amount of longitudinal pull on the extremity, but, as in the case with Buck's traction, it acts more as an immobilizer, and does not actually constitute a great amount of longitudinal pull on the extremity. At any rate, balanced traction is occasionally used in this way, as shown in Figure 2-9.

Russell's Double Traction. Another modification of skin traction used in a balanced setup is Russell's "double" traction. This setup is not nearly as popular as it was in previous years. It does allow for a relatively comfortable traction to be applied without the necessity of using a frame for incorporation of the extremity. As can be seen in Figure 2-11, it probably does not create a complete unit of the lower extremity, as does the regular balanced traction apparatus. Probably it should be considered a variation of Buck's traction rather than as a balanced traction. When one considers it in this light, it seems that it does allow for traction to be applied in the longitudinal direction of the extremity. The desirable effect of slightly flexing the knee is achieved, so that the entire extremity is elevated to a certain extent. Certainly, the traction should be considered more effective than simple Buck's traction.

Thomas Splint with Pierson Attachment. The classical balanced traction, however, requires the use of a pin drilled through the distal femur or through the upper tibia, with a traction bow and a frame consisting of a Thomas traction splint with the so-called Pierson attachment. This classical setup can be suspended in various ways. The author's preference is that shown in Figure 1-5*B*. This allows for a greater range of adjustment and allows for somewhat greater mobility than some of the other balance techniques, in which the latitude of motion is not as great. It would appear that the proper course of action in setting up this traction is to develop a suspension that seems to work well for the individual operator and to use this traction routinely. All operators develop certain favorite points in technique which should be incorporated in their routine practice.

Variations for Children. In children, who are probably the most often treated by balanced traction for fractures of the femur, several variations of technique for balancing the extremity have been developed. One is the cast suspension in which the effective traction is produced by a vectored line, as shown in Figure 1-7*B*. It is not necessary to use a Thomas traction splint with Pierson attachment since the line of pull is straight up at the point of attachment of the pin to the femur. The secondary pull is along the lines of a plaster boot, as shown by line "2," with the vectored traction being along the longitudinal axis of the femur. A slight variation is seen in the "90-90" traction in which the knee is flexed at 90 degrees with pull straight up to a pulley directly overhead (Fig. 2-12). This affords direct pull along the long axis of the femur. The knee is then bent to 90 degrees and a small cast or boot is applied by which the leg can be suspended and stabilized for comfort. This is truly a balanced traction, where the thigh is "balanced" by the pull itself and the leg is "balanced" by an additional pulley and weight setup. This is shown in Figure 2-12*A*.

Fig. 2-12. (Opposite) The various modifications of "90-90" traction for use in femoral fractures in children. In all cases, the traction is applied through a skeletal pin drilled through the distal femur proximal to the epiphyseal plate. The femur is held directly perpendicular to the bed, so that the effect of muscle pull and the effect of gravity can be simultaneously corrected. The modification with the cast suspension *(A)* and with the polyfoam boot traction *(B)* can be used for suspension of the leg. The entire traction setup is applied, *(A and B)*, with the cast and the polyfoam boot merely supplying enough traction to hold the leg up. This is not construed to be a vectored traction. *(Legend continued on page 44.)*

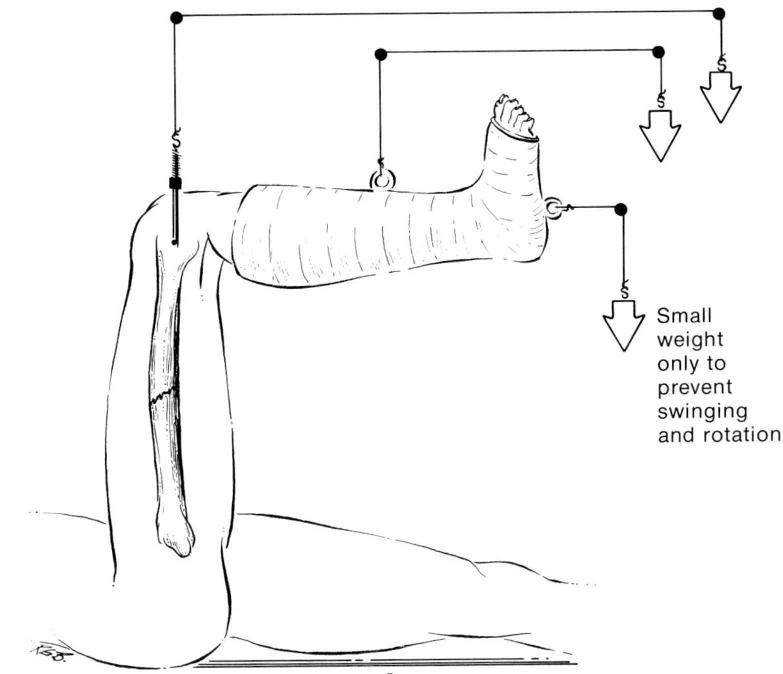
Small
weight
only to
prevent
swinging
and rotation

A

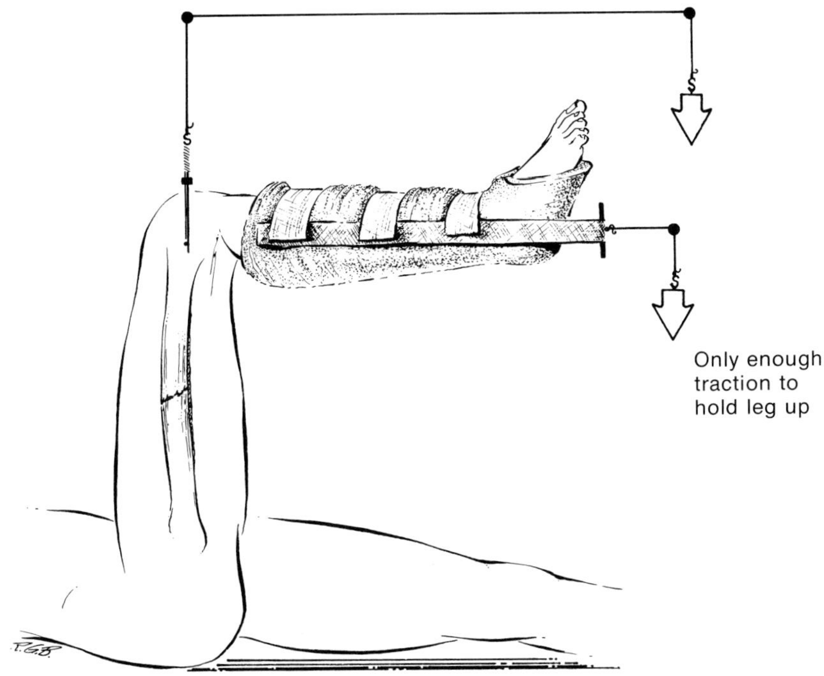
Only enough
traction to
hold leg up

B

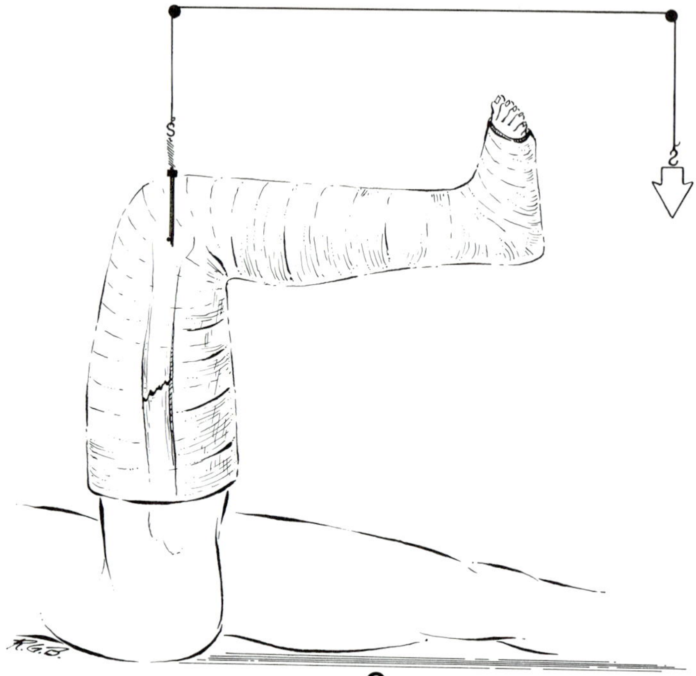

C

Fig. 2-12, continued. (C) The leg is encased in a long-leg plaster cast holding the knee and ankle at right angles, with the pin incorporated in plaster. This is the least desirable method, since pressure phenomena may occur on the posterior calf or at the knee, and may remain unnoticed because of the cast.

Braun-Boehler Frame

The Braun-Boehler frame is a traction frame that supplies support for the lower extremity in instances when traction is needed in the longitudinal axis of the tibia. The appliance shown in Figure 2-13, is fashioned from tubular metal and is adjustable so as to support the lower extremity, with both the hip and knee in approximately 45 degrees of flexion. This may be varied according to the circumstances. The frame lies directly on the bed, usually supported on a wooden platform lying on top of the mattress. The frame is utilized for the application of traction to a transverse pin drilled through either the distal tibia or the os calcis. The frame is particularly useful in the treatment of open fractures of the tibia, since it allows for leaving the lower leg completely exposed and allows for dressing of compound wounds. It also is applied so that the countertraction occurs by the flexion of the knee and is supplied by the thigh resting upon the upper portion of the frame. The traction pin is connected to a traction bow and the rope is passed through a distal pulley so that the traction can be applied directly through the frame itself, without depending upon the externally supplied pulleys and appliances attached to the bed. This makes the Braun-Boehler frame also quite useful in instances in which transportation of the patient is necessary, since the traction apparatus is entirely contained within itself.

The appliance is used for longitudinal traction of femoral fractures when

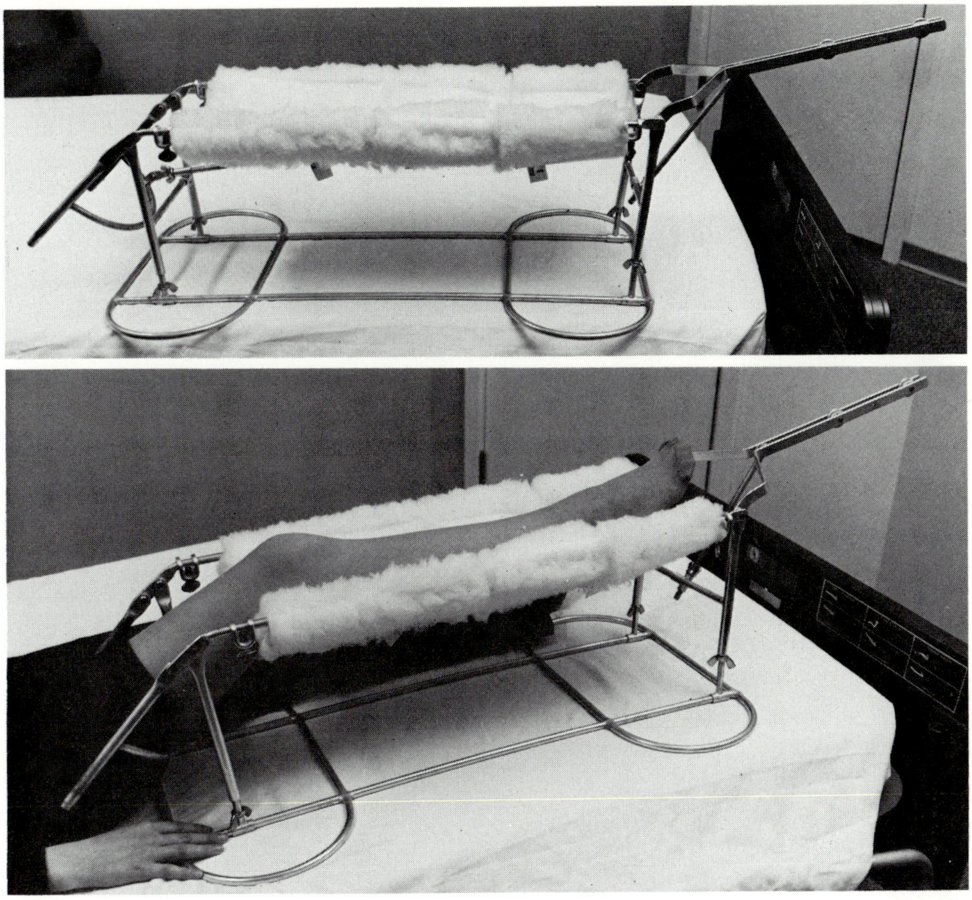

Fig. 2-13. The Braun-Boehler frame. The patient lies recumbent, with the hip and knee both flexed at approximately 45 degrees, on the fabric sling provided with the frame. Traction can be applied through a pin in the distal femur. The line passes over the pulleys on the out-rigger and attaches to a weight, giving a more-or-less mobile traction without the segmental distribution of balanced traction (compare Fig. 1-5). This traction can also be used on the tibia, with countertraction at the flexed knee. A pin is passed through the distal tibia, or even through the os calcis, for the application of continuous traction to the tibia.

transportation is necessary. The pin is placed through the distal femur and traction is applied much as in the balanced traction frame. Treatment of femoral fractures with the frame is not recommended, however. Its use in femoral fractures is recommended basically to a means of transport, and in instances in which it is used only as a temporary device.

In tibial fractures, however, the Braun-Boehler frame is still a very useful mechanism for the application of traction. The leg is maintained in a canvas sling so that posterior angulation does not occur by the effect of gravity. Since the tibia is not surrounded by extremely strong muscles, as is the femur, traction on the tibia to maintain alignment following fractures may be of lesser magnitude than that applied to the femur. It is usually sufficient to apply only a few pounds of traction along the longitudinal axis of the tibia in order to maintain it in position. Application of very much weight usually will result in distraction of fragments. For this reason, the traction *per se* is not enough to overcome the effect of gravity by the "stretching effect," as is seen in femoral fractures. The use of a canvas sling under the leg, to maintain proper alignment and to counteract the effect of gravity, is therefore important in tibial fractures. The traction may then be applied in relatively small amounts only to maintain the length and immobilize the tibia. In this instance, the use of the Braun-Boehler frame is a very satisfactory mechanism for accomplishing immobilization.

Actually, treatment of tibial fractures by traction is not often indicated, since the tibia lends itself well to other types of fixation. When internal fixation is not desirable in the tibia, a simple closed reduction with casting will maintain the position of the fragments. In instances in which this is difficult to do, the application of transfixion pins within the cast will allow the application of casts and will obviate the necessity for traction devices (Fig.2-14). It is when a severe mangling of the extremity occurs, with massive soft tissue damage, that treatment by traction is desirable so that the soft tissue elements of the leg may be left exposed. Here, the Braun-Boehler frame functions admirably and is probably the treatment of choice. It should be noticed, also, that the frame is so designed as to allow for flexion of the knee with the resulting release of the gastroc-soleus musculature, which has its origin above the knee joint. This simple mechanism negates most of the muscle pull from the only muscles that are strong enough to deform tibial fractures. It accounts for the ease with which the position can be maintained in a Braun-Boehler frame with only a small amount of traction.

When fractures in the tibia occur so far distally that insertion of a pin above the ankle joint is not possible, traction by insertion of a relatively large pin through the os calcis is quite permissible. Since the amount of pull that is necessary is not great, a mechanism requiring traction through both the subas-

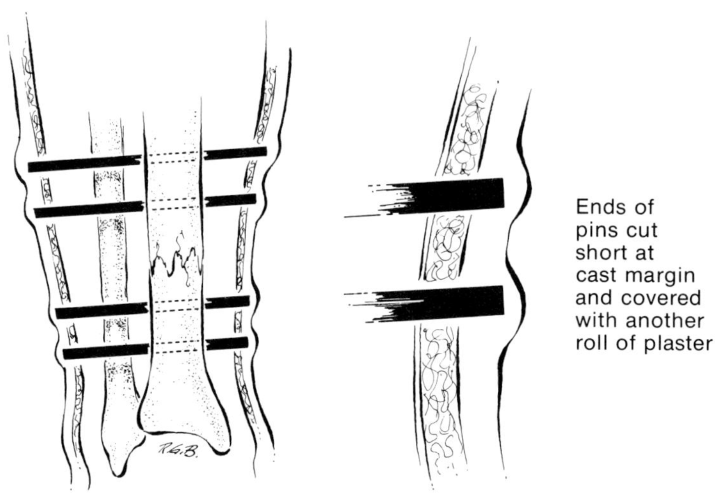

Fig. 2-14. Stabilization of a fracture by incorporating transfixion pins in the cast.

tragalar and the ankle joints is not harmful. Traction through the os calcis may be very satisfactorily applied.

Precautions. A word or two of caution is necessary concerning the use of the Braun-Boehler frame.

There Is No Control Of Rotation. Most of the time, rotation must be assessed visually by the attendant himself. It is very difficult to control rotation in the distal fragment due to the levering effect of the foot, especially when it falls into external rotation. It is extremely important to be aware of this tendency of the distal fragment to externally rotate; care must be taken to prevent the rotatory forces. This can usually be done by placing a small pad or roll underneath the Steinmann pin on the lateral side; this will not interfere with the minimal traction that is being applied. Another mechanism is to simply attach a small cord to the lateral pin and tie it to the frame in order to give a static control of rotation. It should be checked visually daily, and should be checked periodically by x-ray examination as well.

Another important precaution is against the occurrence of equinus deformities in the ankle. They occur almost always when the pin for traction is placed above the ankle. The fixation occurs above the ankle and the foot is allowed to fall freely into equinus, being pulled there by the weight of gravity. Some sort of addition to the frame must be applied to hold the foot in the neutral position. This can be done by means of a small outrigger with a length of stockinett pulled over it, so that the foot rests upon a very soft sling, which prevents the foot from falling into the natural equinus position. The tendency to equinus deformity does not occur when the pin is placed in the os calcis. The pull creates a different fulcrum in the foot which allows the foot to be pulled up into the dorsiflexed position by the traction force itself. When the force is not strong enough, however, it still is necessary to attach an outrigger to the frame to hold the foot up into the neutral, or slightly dorsiflexed, position.

Pin Tracts. A further point of caution concerns care of the pin tracts, particularly when the fracture occurs in the distal tibia and the use of the os calcis is necessary for insertion of the pin. The os calcis, being cancellous in structure, does not allow for a great amount of pull. If it *is* necessary to apply a great amount of traction over a period of time, the use of the os calcis is undesirable. The soft bone will allow for cutting through of the pin, and serious damage may occur. It is likewise important to note that infection is possible in the pin tract, with resultant "ring sequestrum." The ring sequestrum is a sleeve of devitalized bone that forms circumferentially around the pin as it passes through the os calcis. Its formation usually requires surgical removal of the sequestrum and discontinuation of traction by this method. The os calcis does not have a great amount of resistance to infection. The pin applied through the os calcis must be inserted only under the strictest aseptic conditions.

Pin Insertion. It should likewise be pointed out that care must be taken to prevent insertion of the pin through the distal tibia when the fracture extends into the area. Most of the fractures requiring traction with the Braun-Boehler frame are grossly comminuted. It is easy to miss the fracture that extends down into the distal tibia. The area should be carefully examined by roentgenogram prior to the insertion of the pin to be certain that the fracture line does not extend into the area. It is dangerous to insert a pin through a fracture. This procedure invites infection which may migrate through the pin tract to the area of diminished resistance in the fracture line. Infection can be introduced in this area when a pin is inserted through a fracture line.

Pressure Areas. A final word of caution concerns the underside of the leg that must rest on a canvas sling. Since the weight of the leg must rest on a support for long periods of time without moving, one must be very careful to observe frequently for pressure sore formation. It is possible to examine freqently the portion of the leg resting on the sling. When any areas of pressure are identified, vigorous measures must be instituted to prevent their becoming large. For the most part, the treatment of pressure area depends upon shifting the pressure to an area which is uninvolved. The areas in which pressure sores begin to occur require individual analysis and treatment. If the pressure areas become severe, they will constitute an indication for cessation of the Braun-Boehler frame traction and institution of other measures, such as transfixion pin fixation in a cast.

It is preferable to use a sling that is surfaced with one of the artificially made sheepskin pads. Care of the skin must be done periodically to prevent breakdown from maceration, pressure, or both. In spite of these precautions that must be observed, the Braun-Boehler frame offers a very valuable method of management in fractures of the tibia when there is an indication for treatment by traction rather than casting. Open fractures, particularly, are an excellent indication. Traction in the Braun-Boehler frame probably constitutes the most valuable method of treatment of those fractures that have associated severe soft-tissue damage.

Lateral Trochanter. It occasionally becomes necessary to apply a lateral traction to the trochanter of the femur when fractures occur around the hip joint. These may occur as fractures with distortion of the pelvic contour, or they may constitute fractures involving the acetabulum with displacement of the medial wall and intrapelvic protrusion of the femoral head (the so-called central dislocation of the hip). The pull on the lateral trochanter is at right angles to the long axis of the femur, but is associated with traction along the long axis of the femur with a pin through the femoral condyle area. This results in the so-called vectored traction in which the effective line of traction lies somewhere between the lateral and longitudinal traction (demonstrated in Figure 1-6). In other instances, it is merely necessary to apply straight lateral traction to the femur without the longitudinal traction. The extremity is usually suspended in an apparatus so as to make the lateral pull on the trochanter more effective by creating a relative "weightlessness" of the lower extremity. Whatever the ultimate effect of the lateral traction, the attachment of the traction to the trochanter constitutes a major problem. There are multiple types of apparatus that have been devised for attachment to the trochanter, but the selection, from a practical standpoint, usually boils down to two possibilities: the trochanteric "screw," and the "crossed" Steinmann Pins.

The trochanteric "screw" is a screw with large cancellous threads which extends to a ring which protrudes from the skin (Fig. 2-15*A*). This type of fixation is relatively effective, provided the amount of weight is not great. It can be easily seen, however, that there is a tendency for the cancellous threads to pull out through the soft cancellous bone if the weight is excessive. This is a problem particularly in older people with a greater amount of demineralization

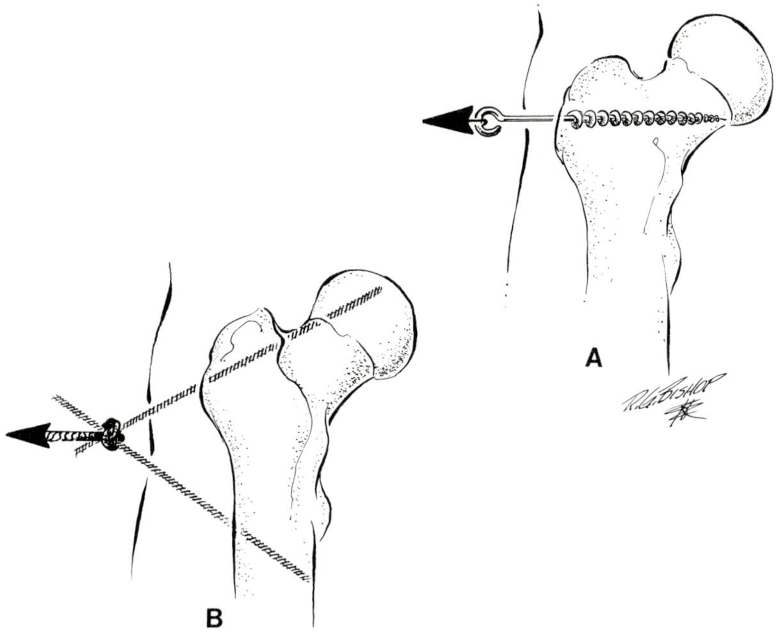

Fig. 2-15. Two types of mechanisms for attachment of traction to the lateral trochanter. *(A)* A heavy cancellous screw. The "lag screw" threads allow for pull at the exposed eye hook without disengagement of the pin from the bone. A large amount of traction is not tolerated with this type of apparatus because of the obvious tendency of the threads to pull out of the soft cancellous bone. The two pins drilled through the upper femur *(B)* are usually placed with the aid of an image intensifier. They must subtend an angle of close to 90 degrees at the point of crossing outside of the skin to give better stability. An angle of about 60 degrees is usually easier to obtain and is acceptable. The traction rope is tied to the site of the crossing of the pins, and traction is applied at right angles to the long axis of the femur. Traction, though, does not usually occur precisely along the long axis of the femoral neck.

of the bone. In younger people, however, lateral pull through a trochanteric screw can be a very effective method. It is somewhat easier to apply than the crossed pin technique.

The crossed pin technique depends upon image intensifier control for proper insertion of the pins so that they are placed at nearly a right angle to one another. As is seen in Figure 2-15*B*, the two pins are drilled through the trochanter and through the upper shaft of the femur so that they cross each other at nearly a right angle, just external to the skin margin. This constitutes a mechanical situation which allows for vigorous pull without detachment, and is probably the method of choice. No matter what mechanism is used in these cases, pull through the trochanter with this type of traction usually is not extremely effective, since the deformity is usually rather great. The pull, no matter how strong, is not enough to dislodge the displaced fragments, particularly when they occur within the pelvis.

When lateral trochanteric traction *is* indicated, however, one of these two methods is recommended.

PELVIC TRACTION

There are two indications for pelvic traction, both with considerable differences in their implications. First, traction may be used for treatment of low back pain. The pelvis acts as the point for attachment of the traction to the body. The pull actually has nothing to do with the pelvis *per se*; rather, it is effective in the lumbar spine. This traction probably should not be called pelvic traction, since it exerts no influence on the pelvis. However, over the years, this traction has become popularly known as "pelvic traction" and, therefore, it will be discussed under that particular heading.

The second type of pelvic traction is that related to fractures of the pelvis itself, even though it does not actually apply traction to the pelvis. This traction is actually applied to the lower extremity or is set up as a pelvic sling, and therefore is not actually a pelvic traction. However, since the ultimate effect is upon the pelvis, it likewise has fallen into this general category.

Finally, traction on the lateral trochanter, as has been previously described, is used basically for fractures through the pelvis itself. It probably can be termed true pelvic traction.

We are faced, then, with misnomers as far as the phrase "pelvic traction" is concerned. However, if we do not concentrate on semantics, but rather discuss the types of traction that are associated with the pelvis *per se*, then the purpose of this discussion will be served.

Low Back Pain

The traction that is applied to the pelvis for the treatment of low back pain actually is traction that is intended for the lumbar spine or, at the very best, for the lumbosacral articulation. The traction that is applied, generally, is applied with the pelvic belt that attaches to the lateral sides of the pelvis by the means of two straps that extend posteriorly, as shown in Figure 2-16. The straps extend down into pulleys and then down to weights for the pull. It is possible to apply from 8 to 10 pounds of weight to either side, making a total of 16 to 20 pounds. It is important that the straps clear the bed and do not touch, since the friction that would occur by impingement of the straps on the mattress would obviate much of the effectiveness of the traction. Pelvic traction should be applied in the so-called Williams position, which was described by Paul Williams some years ago as being of greatest effectiveness for traction to the low back. This position consists of having both knees and hips flexed. The point of greatest importance is the position of the legs from the knees down. The knee-to-ankle position should be parallel to the floor. This results in 30 to 40 degrees of flexion at the knee. From this position, the hips are flexed so that the trunk lies in a reclining position. The hips may then be either further flexed or extended by raising or lowering the head of the bed and increasing or decreasing the inclination of the trunk with respect to the lower extremities. Again, a position of 30 to 45 degrees of flexion in the hips, associated with the previously described position on the lower leg, is generally the position of greatest comfort. In this position, the traction actually serves as little more than a force which holds the pelvis in the "tucked under" position. This is the position, as described by Williams, important in maintaining the greatest diameter of the neural foramina at the lumbosacral level. In instances of acute low back pain,

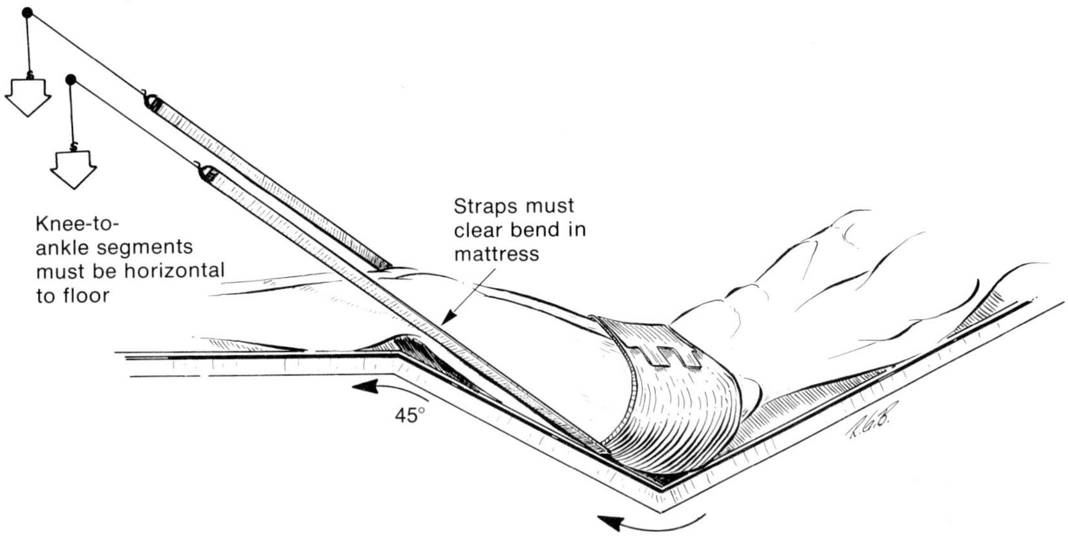

Fig. 2-16. Pelvic traction for low back pain must be properly applied to be effective. The most important factor is position. The hips and knees both must be flexed at approximately 45 degrees. If traction is applied with the patient flat in bed, it will likely make him worse, or it certainly will not be as effective. Note that the pelvic band has attachments of straps posteriorly, so that the traction pulls the pelvis into the flexed or "tucked under" position. The amount of traction need not be great. Only traction that pulls the pelvis into this position with relation to the lumbar spine is effective.

particularly with nerve root irritation, the pelvic traction serves to stabilize the pelvis and to hold it in this flexed position.

This traction may be uncomfortable over long periods of time. The patient is allowed to apply or remove the traction, as necessary, for his comfort. Patients are not instructed to sleep in the traction at night, since this will increase the stiffness and sometimes will increase the amount of pain that they have early in the morning. It is important to note that the pelvic traction should never be applied with the patient lying flat in bed with the hips and knees extended. In this position, the buttocks tend to act as a fulcrum. The pull of the pelvic traction, therefore, causes a hyperextension of the lower lumbar spine and lumbosacral joint, with a considerable increase of pain. The increase of pain is particularly apparent if there is nerve root irritation, since the position of hyperextension narrows the neural foramina and increases the amount of nerve root irritation.

Traction for low back pain is occasionally applied to the lower extremities with Buck's traction, utilizing the sponge rubber traction boot. This is applied to one extremity and sometimes is effective when thus applied. When applied to both extremities simultaneously, however, the patient is quite uncomfortable and is quite immobilized, since both lower extremities are kept entirely still. It will be found that the patient tolerates bilateral Buck's traction very poorly. This traction is not nearly as effective as traction with the pelvic apparatus.

The same implications exist, as far as position is concerned, with the bilateral Buck's traction as with pelvic traction. The traction must be applied in the Williams position with moderate flexion of the hips and knees. Otherwise, the symptoms will be made more severe, and the effects of the traction will become deleterious rather than helpful (Fig. 2-9).

Pelvic Fractures

As mentioned in the introduction to this section, most of the traction that is applied for fractures of the pelvis cannot be called truly "pelvic traction," but rather should be called traction that is used in the treatment of pelvic fractures. For instance, the most commonly used pelvic traction is the pelvic sling. This is demonstrated in Figure 2-17*A*. It is a canvas sling that is passed under the pelvis. The sling is attached to a spreader bar which maintains the walls of the sling in a nearly parallel position so that no undue lateral pressure occurs on the trochanters. The entire pelvis is encased in a single sling that immobilizes the pelvis and converts it into a single mechanical entity. This traction does not do much to reduce existing fractures. It does convert the pelvis into a single unit so that movement of the remainder of the body can occur with less pain. It is well known that most fractures of the pelvis will heal almost in spite of treatment that is rendered, since the innominate bones are made up principally of cancellous bone. During the healing stage, however, there is considerable pain with movement. It has been demonstrated that with a pelvic sling the patient will be much more comfortable because he can move the lower extremities and can move the upper part of his torso without causing movement through the pelvic fractures. This traction is applied in a single area by the use of a spreader bar, and the amount of weight is usually enough to provide an almost weightless condition for the pelvis itself. In other words, when the pelvic sling has been applied properly, the hand can be passed between the buttocks and the bed with little difficulty, indicating that the buttocks are barely touching the bed. The pelvic sling is usually applied until the patient has become reasonably comfortable and until the fractures have adhered enough so that he can be mobilized in some type of canvas corset. As previously indicated, the pelvic sling does not constitute a definitive treatment of pelvic bone fractures; rather, it creates a stabilizing or immobilizing effect on these fractures.

When separation of the symphysis pubis has occurred and a compressive force is indicated, the pelvic sling is converted into a "crossed compression traction" setup. This is demonstrated in Figure 2-17*B*. The two ends of the pelvic sling are detached from the spreader bar previously used in the pelvic sling setup; each is attached to a pulley lying on the opposite side of the patient. This, then, allows for a compressive effect from side to side and does have a definitive effect on separated fractures, particularly in the anterior pelvic ring. The amount of traction can be varied according to the amount of compression force used. The weightless condition of the pelvis cannot be created, as it is with a plain pelvic sling, since it is impossible to apply this much traction to either side of the sling. On the other hand, the sling does have a supportive or immobilizing effect, since the compressive force carries with it a certain amount of pelvic support. The main disadvantage of this traction is that it causes considerable pressure over the trochanteric region; most of these

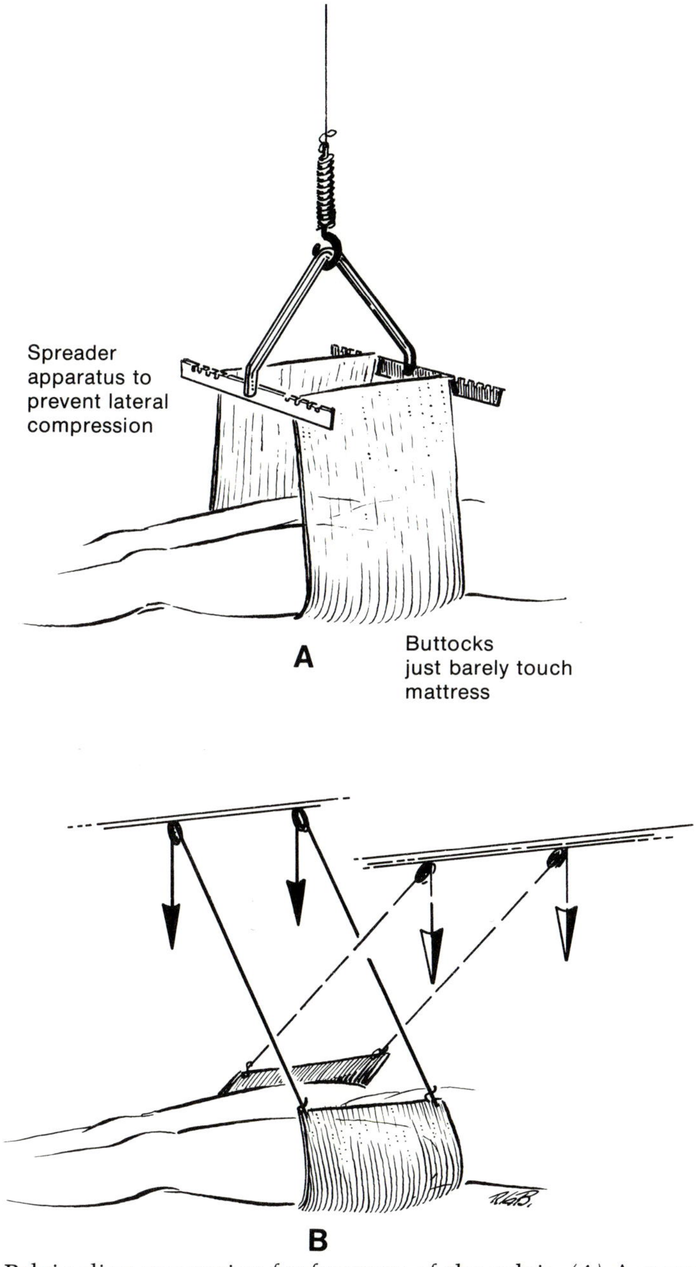

Fig. 2-17. Pelvic sling suspension for fractures of the pelvis. *(A)* A suspension of the pelvis without an attempt at compression. The sling is suspended by means of a large metal frame, and weight is applied so that the pelvis is largely counterbalanced and becomes, to a certain extent, "weightless." Movement can then occur without moving the pelvic fragments. *(B)* The method for applying compression when there has been separation of the anterior pelvic ring, particularly at the symphysis pubis. The suspension in this type of traction is not as great, but is effective to a certain extent. This suspension compresses the pelvis from side to side to correct any diastasis that may have occurred. Pain developing at pressure points over the trochanters is unavoidable; it will often limit the duration of time that compression traction is useful.

patients will complain of soreness developing over the trochanters. Some even develop a severe trochanteric bursitis which may necessitate discontinuation of traction. It is possible to use compressive traction for a week or so until the fragments have been brought into better alignment, and then to change to a simple pelvic sling, if the trochanters have become sore enough to warrant discontinuation of compressive traction.

When there has been a cephalad displacement of the hemipelvis on one side or the other due to associated fractures of the anterior and posterior positions of the pelvic ring, it is necessary to apply balanced traction through the femur to reduce the displaced hemipelvis. This traction is applied with a pin through the distal femur and a balanced traction frame, as has been previously described. A tremendous amount of weight is required to cause a reduction of cephalad displacement of the hemipelvis; often it is found that even though tremendous amounts of weight are applied, the pelvic displacement cannot be reduced. This is particularly true if the fracture occurs long before the traction is first applied. If traction through the femur is applied relatively soon after the injury, however, a considerable improvement in the cephalad displacement can be achieved. Again, the amount of weight used must be considerable (exceeding 40 or 50 pounds). Once the traction has been decreased, it is necessary to continue the traction over a period of several weeks for the fractures to heal enough to maintain position.

This traction has one serious disadvantage; it usually results in symptoms referable to the hip joint, which is considerably stretched in the process of applying the pelvic traction. Prolonged traction through the hip joint will result in stretching of the capsule. There have been reported instances of diminished blood supply to the femoral head from stretching of the capsular vessels which serve the head. It is, therefore, recommended that when any weight is applied to the femur with traction through the hip joint to the pelvis, this traction be maintained only for a relatively short period of time and be reduced as soon as it is felt that the fracture is stable. Serial roentgenograms that reveal inferior subluxation of the hip joint should be an indication for discontinuation of traction, or at least for a marked reduction in the amount of weight applied.

The application of lateral trochanter traction, described in the last section, is a definitive treatment for fractures of the hemipelvis that involve the acetabulum. For the most part, this traction is used with the so-called central dislocation of the hip in which the femoral head is driven through the medial wall of the acetabulum into the pelvis. Considerable traction is required for reduction of the fragment. Though it is possible to withdraw the femoral head from the intrapelvic position back into a more nearly normal relationship with the roof of the acetabulum, it is rarely possible to achieve reduction of the inner wall of the acetabulum and associated pelvic fractures. If the displacement is great with marked distortion of the acetabular wall, consideration should be given to more definitive surgical reconstruction of the acetabular architecture. The reader is referred to extensive material in the orthopedic literature concerning the indications for this type of surgery.

When lateral traction is applied, however, it is necessary to use the crossed Steinmann pin technique described in the last section. The amount of weight necessary to move the intrapelvic protrusion of the femoral head will be considerable; the amount of traction that can be applied through a trochanteric screw is not likely to be great enough to have the desired effect. In most significantly displaced pelvic fractures, the effect of any traction in securing reduction of the fractures, *per se*, is likely to be disappointing. The innominate bone is almost entirely cancellous; fractures that are displaced are likely to be relatively stable in the displaced position because of the architecture of the pelvis. When one seeks, however, only to withdraw the femoral head from an intrapelvic position by lateral cross pin traction, or when one seeks to supply immobilization and stabilization in fractures that are minimally displaced, or when one seeks to immobilize fractures that are displaced but in satisfactory position, then the results of traction applied for pelvic fractures are satisfactory.

3 Casting and Splinting—General Considerations

The oldest form of treatment of fractures is external immobilization. Since the earliest writings on medical care, broken extremities have been treated by attachment of some type of splinting device. This helps to immobilize the fractured bone contained within the extremity. While there are some distinct advantages to external immobilization, there are disadvantages that make it a form of treatment that is indicated only in selected instances.

ADVANTAGES

The most obvious advantage to this type of external immobilization is that it is nonoperative. It does not require an open incision, thus precluding the possibility of postoperative wound infection. Being nonoperative, the external immobilization may not require a general anesthetic; many of the complications associated with operative intervention and general anesthesia are prevented. Along with the nonoperative advantages of external immobilization is included an economic aspect; it is less expensive. External immobilization can be done without hospitalization, and it certainly does not require the operating room fee and the other expenses associated with open reduction. A final advantage is the fact that dynamic correction can be established with external immobilization, in certain cases. This can be one of the major advantages to this type of treatment. Splints can be fashioned with dynamic features such as elastic pull straps; fractures can be corrected with gradual wedging of the cast, and other forms of dynamic correction can be used that are actually therapeutic. Many of these features make external immobilization by casting or splinting advantageous, and will make it the treatment of choice in certain cases.

LIMITATIONS

Just as there are certain advantages to casting and splinting in the treatment of fractures, there are certain limitations to this form of immobilization. First, the immobilization is not as complete. The interposition of soft tissue between the supporting or immobilizing device and the fractured bone renders the immobilization less effective, since motion can take place within this soft-tissue sleeve. It is, however, possible to improve the efficiency of immobilization by observing certain principles for positioning the extremity at the time of casting. These features will be discussed in some detail later in the chapter.

The second important limitation to remember is that *holding* features of external immobilization are better than the correction features. It is not often possible to secure a great amount of correction with a simple casting procedure unless some dynamic feature is installed into the fixation device. This includes the use of springs, rubberbands, and other such appliances to help correct certain deformities. This is not usually applicable to acute fractures, though it is possible to wedge the cast in order to improve position, particularly when angulation is present. When one attempts to *correct* the position by application of a cast, the most important complication to be avoided is the occurrence of pressure areas. When one attempts to correct an angulation and hold it in plaster in the corrected position against resistance (such as may occur in attempting to correct a green stick fracture without breakthrough the other cortex), pressure areas will develop at the point where the cast is pushed against the extremity. Attempting to hold fractures which require some resistance for correction is most dangerous. Casts of this nature should be applied only with great caution.

Pressure points of all sorts must be avoided in the application of external splinting devices. This is particularly true on the margins of metallic or plastic splints, which will cut into the soft tissue if wrapped too tightly. Certain bony prominences must be protected by adequate padding in order to prevent the development of pressure areas over them. Examples include the head of the fibula, the malleoli of the ankle, and the epicondyles of the distal humerus.

In all these instances, an improperly applied cast can cause complete destruction of soft tissue by causing pressure between the cast and the underlying bone; an indolent ulcer may develop that could be extremely difficult to heal. Prevention of these pressure areas depends not only upon adequate padding over the areas, but also upon adequate molding of the cast in an effort to secure fit. By molding the plaster as it dries, following the exact contour of the extremity, one can form the cast so that it fits the bony prominences quite well. Pressure areas can, in this way, be prevented. Pressure areas, likewise, are much easier to prevent if the cast is well fitting so that no motion occurs between the cast and the extremity; many pressure areas begin as friction injuries at a point of rubbing between the cast and the bony prominence of the extremity.

INSURING EFFECTIVENESS

Mention should be made of various measures to increase the effectiveness of external casting and splinting devices, since the immobilization is not as complete as it is with internal fixation. By utilizing these various principles, casting and splinting devices may be used effectively to immobilize fractures of the extremities.

Position

The importance of position in the application of casts to acute fractures cannot be overemphasized. It is well known that the line of muscle pull acts as a deforming factor in many of these fractures. It, therefore, follows that if the position is made so that the deforming muscle pull is counteracted, the fracture is likely to be much more stable, a good example is shown in Figure 3-1*A*.

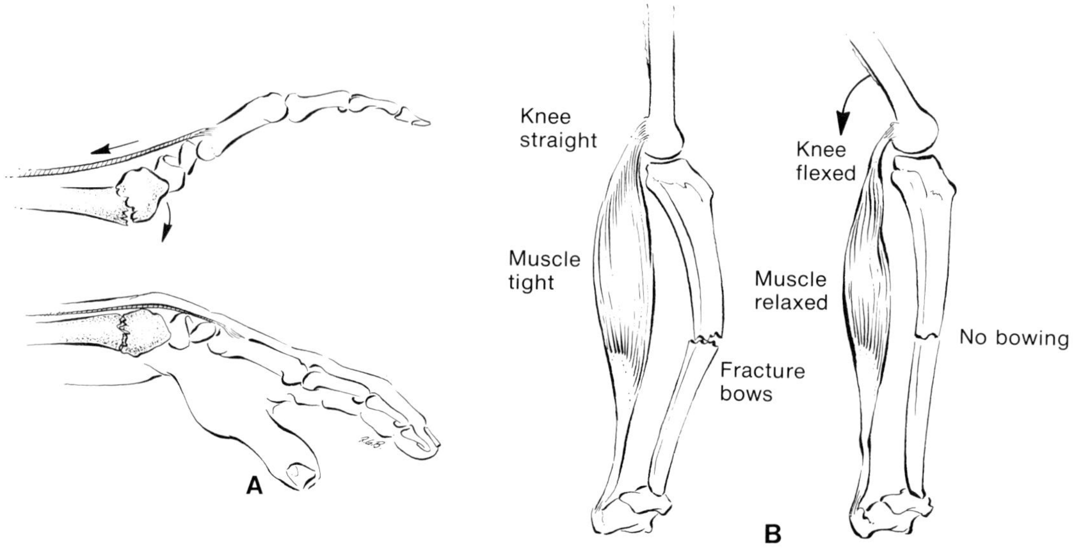

Fig. 3-1. The effect of position in maintaining reduction of a fracture. *(A)* A fracture of the radius that is dorsally displaced is maintained in the dorsally displaced position by action of the extensor tendons, which bowstring to keep the distal fragment in the dorsally displaced position. Reduction can be obtained manually, but it is necessary to keep the wrist in flexion in order to decrease the mechanical advantage of the extensor tendons, thereby maintaining reduction of the fracture. *(B)* A similar condition occurring in the tibia, wherein the bowstringing effect from the tight gastroc-soleus group results in anterior bowing of the fracture of the tibia with the knee straight. With the knee flexed, however, the gastroc-soleus muscle loses its mechanical advantage and becomes relaxed, so that the fracture is made stable. This accounts in part for the necessity of maintaining a fracture of the tibia in a long-leg cast with the knee in flexion.

In fractures of the distal radius, the distal fragment is likely to be angulated dorsally by overpull of the extensor musculature. If, after the fracture is reduced, the fracture line is otherwise stable, the likelihood of loss of position at the fracture site is much less if the wrist is put up in flexion. By putting the wrist up in flexion, the effect of the extensor pull is obviated; the extensors are put up in a position where the mechanical advantage has been diminished. Many instances are seen in Colles' fractures where reduction is lost and dorsal angulation is resumed in the distal fragment, all because of poor position in the immobilization device. In almost all instances, a Colles' fracture can be put up in flexion; in flexion it should be stable enough so that reduction is likely to be maintained.

A second illustration of the importance of position in controlling muscle pull is that of fractures of the mid-shaft of the tibia, which tend to bow anteriorly because of the pull of the gastroc-soleus group. These fractures must be maintained in position by the application of a cast which keeps the knee in marked flexion, decreasing the mechanical advantage of the gastroc-soleus group. This position prevents the bowstringing effect that these muscles have; it prevents anterior angulation at the fracture site (Fig. 3-1*B*).

Along with the effect of muscle pull, the *type* of fracture that has occurred is of extreme importance. An example is shown in Figure 3-2. A fracture of the posterior malleolus of the ankle results in a very unstable situation, unless the ankle is put up with the foot in dorsiflexion. In this position, the capsular attachments to the fracture pull the fracture down into anatomic position, and the fracture can quite easily be maintained. Failure to put the ankle up in marked dorsiflexion, however, will result in failure to maintain position of the bones posteriorly, and will result in loss of stability of the posterior aspect of the ankle.

One final point should be mentioned from the standpoint of position. Awkward positions of the extremity necessary to hold a fracture in position are tolerated for short periods of time, but the extremity should not be left in these awkward and grotesque positions over a long period. Contractural phenomena may occur. An example may be the application of a cast in marked inversion of the foot to prevent distraction of a medial malleolus fracture. This position may be satisfactory for a period of 5 to 6 weeks. After the extremity is left in position for that period, the fracture will have begun to heal. Enough healing will have taken place to make the site more stable. A more nearly normal anatomic position can be restored and the cast reapplied in this more acceptable position. Leaving the extremity in abnormal positions for a protracted period of time results in a marked lengthening of the convalescence and a marked increase in the difficulty of rehabilitation once the fracture has healed and the cast has been removed.

Extent

The extent of the immobilization device is a second consideration for insuring effectiveness of the device. The old axiom that dictates the joint above and below a fracture be immobilized is a valid one. It may be necessary also, to

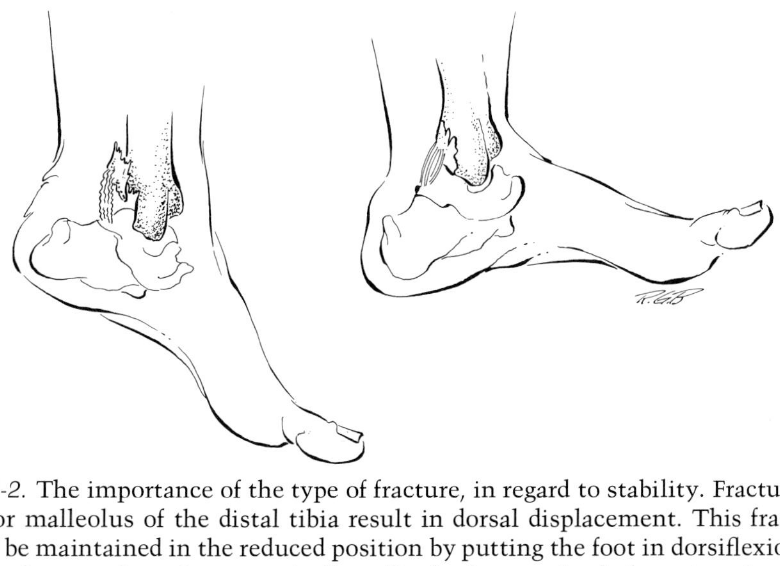

Fig. 3-2. The importance of the type of fracture, in regard to stability. Fractures of the posterior malleolus of the distal tibia result in dorsal displacement. This fracture can usually be maintained in the reduced position by putting the foot in dorsiflexion, which tightens the capsule and automatically pulls the fracture back down into its anatomic position. The capsular attachment makes this reduction possible.

immobilize the joints on either side of a fracture in order to relieve muscle pull and to provide increased stability. It is necessary to include the joint above and below the fracture to extend the immobilizatioin to include both ends of the bone.

Motion in a joint formed by the end of the bone containing a fracture results in motion through the bone and, therefore, through the fracture site. An example of this is seen in fractures of the tibia. With fractures occurring through the distal tibia, it is often tempting to try to immobilize the fracture with a short-leg cast so that the knee motion can be maintained. However, the gastroc–soleus muscle group attaches above the knee joint, but its insertion is through the Achilles tendon attaching to the os calcis. Motions in this muscle, therefore, result in movements through the fracture site. Immobilization cannot be maintained as long as this muscle is allowed to move without restriction. Motion through the knee also causes minor motion at the fracture site; this adds to the instability of the fracture and incompleteness of the immobilization.

Another factor that would preclude treating a lower tibial fracture with a short-leg cast is rotation. If a fracture occurs through the entire shaft of the bone and a short-leg cast is applied, even though well molded, the distal fragment and the remainder of the extremity distal to the fracture are converted into a single unit. The cylindrical nature of the cast above the fracture site allows rotary motion of the foot, resulting in rotation through the fracture site with a shearing motion that will preclude healing. Extension of this cast above the knee, with the knee in 45 or 50 degrees of flexion, will combat these factors. It will (1) prevent motion at the knee with resulting motion in the tibia, which forms one of the articular surfaces of the knee. It will (2) prevent motion of the gastroc-soleus group and, therefore, prevent stress on the fracture site by contractions of this muscle acting through the fracture. Finally, it will (3) prevent rotation by immobilizing the knee joint and creating a single unit of the entire extremity rather than just of the distal fragment (Fig. 3-3),

The same features can be seen in fractures through the distal femur. Again, particularly with fracture-dislocations through the distal femoral epiphysis in adolescent patients, there is a temptation to reduce the badly angulated fracture and immobilize it in a long-leg cast extending up to the groin.

The same factors are active as in the fracture of the tibia. Immobilization cannot be obtained in this manner. Motions through the hip joint will result in a certain amount of motion in the proximal fragment of the femur, with disruption of stability at the fracture site. The hamstring muscles, which attach above the hip joint and below the knee joint, likewise will produce motion through the fracture site if they are allowed to contract, or if muscle pull is allowed by flexion at the hip joint. Finally, rotation cannot be controlled with a long-leg cast. The distal fragment is converted with the remainder of the extremity distal to it, into a single unit. The cylindrical shape of a cast that extends only to the groin allows rotation through the fracture site. The application of a hip spica cast to immobilize the hip joint obviates all three of these factors. Adequate immobilization can be obtained by nothing less than incorporation in a hip spica cast.

A final illustration concerns the Colles' fracture. It has been pointed out that the Colles' fracture is much more stable with the wrist in flexion; this reestab-

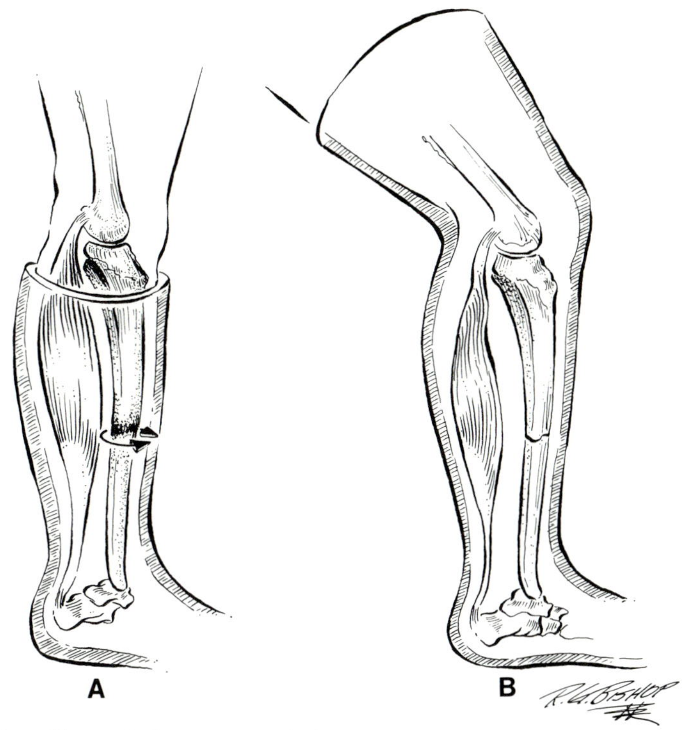

Fig. 3-3. The effect of the extent of the cast is demonstrated in a fracture of the mid-shaft of the tibia. *(A)* A short-leg cast that does not control the knee joint not only allows for tightening of the gastroc-soleus group, with a tendency to anterior bowing of the tibia, but also the cast and the lower extremity, with the foot encased, act as a single unit, allowing rotation at the fracture site. With the ankle at right angles and the cast extending only up past the fracture site, but not above the knee joint, the foot acts as a fulcrum, which is a powerful mechanical factor in causing rotation. Similarly, knee-joint motion allows motion of the proximal fragment by its contiguous location. *(B)* In contrast, the long-leg cast with the knee flexed results in loosening of the gastrocnemius muscle, which relieves the bowstringing effect. Similarly, rotation is controlled by flexion of the knee and 0-degree position at the ankle, thus giving two points of fixation from the standpoint of rotation. The long-leg cast likewise restricts motion at the knee.

lishes a more sound mechanical situation at the fracture site. However, as long as pronation and supination are allowed to occur unchecked, there still occurs a shearing force at the fracture site, which results in loss of position. A small amount of flexion and extension motion in the elbow does not interfere with stability. However, since the control of supination and pronation is important, it is necessary to immobilize these fractures in some type of cast or splint—one that will control these various features and still maintain the flexed position at the wrist. Many surgeons employ the so-called suger-tong splint as the best method of fulfilling these needs. The sugar-tong splint consists of a long plaster splint molded from the dorsum of the hand at the level of the proximal joints of the fingers, over the dorsum of the wrist, forearm, and around the dorsum of the elbow to extend onto the volar side, extending down again to the proximal flexion crease of the palm (see Fig. 6-3). By putting the sugar-tong splint on, with the wrist in the flexed position and the forearm in a neutral position, supination and pronation are controlled very nicely. A small amount of inconsequential motion is still allowed at the elbow. Only by including the elbow in the immobilization apparatus can complete and adequate immobilization of the fracture occur.

Contact

It has been mentioned earlier that molding of the cast is extremely important if one is to secure adequate immobilization of the fracture, and, at the same time, prevent pressure areas from developing (Fig. 3-4). The technique for molding the plaster during the setting period will be discussed later. By stroking and rubbing the plaster into the irregular contours of the extremity, it can be applied in a form-fitting manner, so that support is much improved and the bony prominences are better protected from pressure. The use of adequate padding is essential. While the padding over the shaft areas of the extremity is not as important, care must be taken to provide adequate soft padding over bony prominences, such as the head of the fibula.

One must, particularly in well-molded casts, be very cautious about circulation in the extremity. Since the cast is circumferential, it is very easy for swelling in the cast to have a constrictive effect on the underlying blood vessels, resulting in vascular insufficiency to the extremity distal to the point of constriction. It is wise to split casts applied to acute fractures of extremities immediately postoperatively, in order that swelling may occur without resulting in circumferential constriction. A segment of cast only 1 or 2 cm. in width can be removed, for instance, from the anterior aspect of a short-leg cast, extending from the toe margin up to the upper margin, without jeopardizing the effectiveness of the cast. This allows enough freedom so that circumferen-

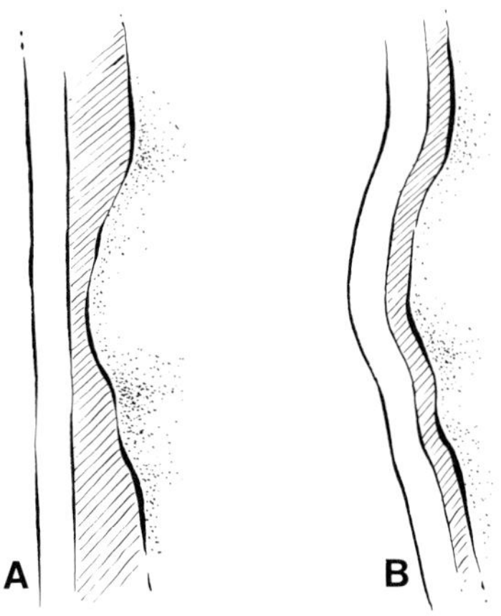

Fig. 3-4. The effect of molding in the prevention of pressure areas. *(A)* The cast has not been molded, and consequently the area of bony prominence is subjected to abnormal pressure by the side of the cast. The cast is suspended upon this one area of prominence. *(B)* Molding has been done so that there is an even pressure in all areas. Molding is important over all areas underlying a cast, but it is of particular importance over bony prominences.

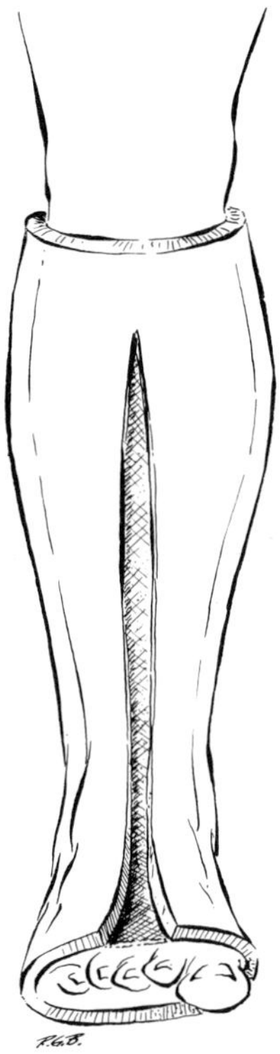

Fig. 3-5. After the short-leg cast is applied, it is often split to allow for postoperative swelling and to allow an area for proper spreading of the cast, if necessary. A 1-cm.-wide strip is removed from the tip of the cast up to the proximal portion, but not including the last 2 or 3 cm. of the cast. By leaving this bridge, the cast maintains its stability, but the area in which swelling might occur is underneath the split area.

tial constriction is not likely to occur (Fig. 3-5). The cast is split more efficiently when fresh, from a mechanical viewpoint. As swelling occurs, the cast can be mechanically spread; as the swelling subsides, the cast can be compressed back against the extremity to maintain effective immobilization.

Even though most of the cast padding material now in use (sheet wadding and other proprietary preparations) is somewhat flimsy and conceivably may tear if swelling becomes a problem, one cannot always count on spontaneous disruption of the padding. Therefore, when the cast has been split and when marked swelling occurs, it may be necessary not only to spread the cast slightly, but also to cut the sheet wadding to prevent circumferential constriction caused from the cast or its padding. It is important, then, to follow the patient carefully; as the swelling subsides, the cast may be tightened. An extremely loose cast will not only fail to immobilize the fracture properly, but also may even have a deleterious effect due to its weight and shifting position. It might be mentioned that the sugar-tong splint, previously described in treatment of Colles' fractures, is attached with loosely applied elastic bandages so that swelling may occur by separation of the two sides of the sugar tong. At the same time, however, as shrinking of the extremity occurs and swelling subsides, the splints are still held in close apposition with the extremity.

The cast or splint that does not have close contact with the contours of the extremity usually does not give adequate immobilization. Therefore, one must be careful that appliances, whether cast or splint, fit the contours of the extremity perfectly, and that allowances are made for swelling and shrinking of the extremity. Very careful supervision of the patient's immobilization in external fixation devices is mandatory if one is to maintain adequate fixation and to avoid the complications previously described.

Pin Incorporation

The use of pin incorporation in casts provides a technique whereby the effectiveness of immobilization by casting can often be markedly improved. Pins may be drilled above and below the fracture site for incorporation into the plaster, as in Figure 2-14, or may be drilled across the fracture site and combined with external immobilization. This provides a "middle ground" between true external immobilization and open operative fixation. An incision is not made, though the skin is entered with the fixation pins.

The introduction of the pin is done under aseptic conditions, using either a manually or mechanically driven drill. Usually, two pins are placed above and below the fracture site and are left protruding through the skin on either side. The fracture is then reduced and the plaster-of-paris cast is applied, incorporating and stabilizing the pins.

Transfixion pin fixation, with incorporation in the cast, is particularly useful in comminuted fractures of the tibia in which shortening occurs. Because of the lack of stability and the comminution at the fracture site, the continuous muscle pull results in a collapse at the fracture site with obvious shortening of the extremity. It is not possible to hold these fractures by means of a cast alone. The shortening will occur even with the cast. Once the pins are drilled through the bone above and below the fracture site and incorporated into plaster, the distance between the pins is maintained by the solidarity of the plaster, and length can be maintained. The pins are usually cut off and bent over as they emerge from the plaster on either side; additional plaster is applied to hold them in place. This securely fixes the fracture, and excellent immobilization is achieved. With badly comminuted fractures in which shortening is a problem, transfixation with pins and incorporation in plaster probably constitute the treatment of choice.

For more detailed information concerning the exact technique of transfixion pin fixation and application of the cast, the reader is referred to textbooks on fracture treatment.

4 Plaster-of-Paris Casts

Probably nothing in the history of orthopaedic surgery has had as great an impact on the treatment of fractures as has the development of plaster of paris. First described by a Flemish army surgeon, plaster of paris gained quick and widespread popularity because it opened broad new concepts in the treatment of fractures of the extremities. Prior to this, the basic form of treatment following closed reduction was support of the fracture by application of an external splint. These splints were sometimes quite elaborate. They were composed of material that followed the contour of the extremity reasonably well; however, they left much to be desired both from the standpoint of fit and from the standpoint of ease of application. The fact that these externally applied devices were not adaptable to the contour of the extremity rendered them quite inefficient in holding fractures once they had been reduced. It was the development of the concept of the circumferential rigid casement that added a new dimension. Not only could the plaster be molded to fit the extremity exactly, but also it could be molded and held while the plaster dried in such a way that the desired position of the extremity could be maintained. This obviously allowed a much wider latitude in treatment techniques. As other methods of application, such as the incorporation of transfixion pins, have been developed, these concepts have broadened even further. At present, it is difficult for the average orthopaedist to conceive of treating fractures of the extremities without using plaster of paris. Along with the use of plaster in the formation of circumferential casements (casts), its use in forming splints has likewise offered a much more exacting immobilization for fractures not requiring fully circumferential casts.

The use of plaster of paris has become an integral part of the armamentarium of the physician treating injuries to the extremities. A thorough knowledge of the methods of application of plaster immobilization is imperative if one is to achieve any expertise in management of these conditions.

CHEMISTRY AND ACTION

Basically, the plaster used today is a hemihydrate of calcium sulfate, which has the property of uniting with water in a chemical reaction that produces gypsum. Gypsum "sets" in the position maintained during the "setting" process and becomes quite hard, but relatively light weight. As it dries the plaster becomes somewhat brittle, but still maintains enough strength to support the average extremity quite well, if properly applied.

This plaster powder is used to impregnate rolls or strips of a crinoline-type material which has been impregnated with a starch compound to make it stiff.

When the plaster-of-paris powder is caught in the meshes of the crinoline, the entire roll of crinoline is dipped into water to commence the chemical reaction which transfers the plaster to gypsum. By having the plaster thus enmeshed in crinoline the roll of plaster easily can be applied circumferentially to the extremity. The crinoline, further, acts as a unit or a reinforcement mechanism that allows the plaster to be held in the desired shape while the setting process occurs. Likewise, these rolls of wet crinoline become limp enough to allow for careful molding; as the plaster sets, the pliable crinoline can be molded nicely to follow any desired contour. Once setting has occurred, the crinoline acts as a reinforcement mesh, much in the same manner that steel mesh is used in concrete to prevent cracking and to give better lateral stability.

It is possible to develop circular casts that are quite thin, but that have considerable lateral strength due to: (1) the strength of the plaster material and its crinoline mesh, and (2) the inherent strength of a tubular structure. The chemical reaction which develops gypsum from plaster of paris is an exothermic reaction; the cast becomes quite hot during the setting stage. Its transfer into a rigid compound can be gauged by the sensation of heat. Once the heat of chemical reaction is felt with the applying hands, the operator knows that the cast soon will be solid. As the reaction becomes complete, the exothermic reaction subsides. The heat quickly dissipates, leaving the plaster quite moist, cold, and clammy.

Complete drying of the plaster requires a good many hours, since it it necessary for the water to evaporate to leave a totally dry, rigid cast. While the reaction is not reversible, wetting the cast will make it soft and cause it to fragment. Occasionally, it will break if it is allowed to become wet and stay wet for any length of time. The susceptibility to wetness, however, is not so great as to preclude occasionally cleaning the surface of the cast with a damp cloth, but it *does* preclude immersion in water.

CHARACTERISTICS OF PLASTER OF PARIS

Consistency

Many commercial manufacturers of plaster vary the consistency by varying the chemical formula, particularly with the use of additives.

Creamy. Some plaster is quite creamy. Such a plaster is represented by Gypsona. Gypsona tends to be somewhat whiter and faster setting, but tends to be softer. It does not have the hard consistency when dry as does coarser plaster, since additives to the plaster decrease its strength after drying. Creamy plaster, however, does make a very beautiful cast because it is so smooth. It can be made into a very smooth, perfectly contoured cast by massage during the setting stage.

Plaster such as this has a great advantage because of its fast setting properties in situations such as the application of corrective casts to club feet in infants. The rapidity with which setting occurs is quite valuable; the fact that the plaster is not quite as strong is of little consequence. This plaster tends to become extremely soft when wet. In infants with club feet, it may be soaked off by the mother at home the night before bringing the child into the office. Skin care may be given and the skin may be allowed to dry before the change of casts.

Creamy plaster is often used for gauntlet casts for the hand and other small casts which do not require great strength, but in which smoothness and lightness are of primary value.

Coarse. Other plaster is more coarsely made. This occurs because certain additives tend to alter the drying properties of the plaster; also, coarser meshed crinoline is used. These plasters are much more durable, stronger, and much more resistant to wetting than the creamier types. They are somewhat slower in drying, though plasters may have additives that allow extremely fast drying, when desired. Between these two extremes of creamy and coarse plaster, there are as many variations as there are manufacturers. The physician will discover one type of plaster that more nearly suits his general needs, and will settle on that plaster for his every day use. The other specialty plasters may then be kept in reserve for special occasions, when they arise.

Strength

The strength of plaster is varied by alteration of the chemical formula, particularly with the addition of certain resins. As mentioned above, there is some difference in the strength of the plaster as related to its consistency. Certain preparations are available commercially which have resins added that yield a very strong and extremely water-resistant cast. An example is a product manufactured by Johnson and Johnson and distributed under the trade name Zoroc. This plaster has added resin that not only makes the plaster stronger and more water resistant, but also makes it faster drying. Zoroc is more expensive than plain plaster, and therefore is saved for occasions when the necessity for strength, durability, and water resistance overshadows the additional cost.

Position. There are factors besides chemical additives that influence the strength of plaster casts. The position of the extremity is of considerable importance. As an example, the long-leg cast with the knee bent at 90 degrees is not nearly so stable at the knee as is the cast that is made with the knee in only slight flexion. This is because the leverage placed on a knee flexed at 90 degrees requires greater structural strength at the 90-degree bend. For this reason, certain casts, such as long-leg casts, should have structural splints added to the sides to improve strength. The addition of extra layers of plaster and crinoline base provides additional lines of reinforcement.

Other examples of stress points are upper and lower margins of hyperextension body jackets. Considerable stress is applied to them by the attempts of the torso to flex in the cast. Undue stress is applied to the upper and lower margins of the anterior portion of the cast, which presses against the sternum and the pubis. These areas of the cast must be much stronger than the area lying over the abdomen, for instance, which is relatively free from mechanical stress. Care must be taken to give greater thickness to plaster and to apply splints (which in themselves increase the mechanical stability of the cast) where unusual mechanical strain is likely to occur.

Molding. Another important factor which has great importance from the standpoint of strength of the cast is molding. While cylinder casts have a great amount of inherent strength by virtue of the mechanical stability of the cylinder shape, they can be greatly improved by careful molding over the exact contour of the extremity. The variations in the roundness of the contour can be reproduced by molding the cast over the contour of the extremity while the plaster is drying. This greatly increases the mechanical strength of the cylinder by virtue of making it more nearly form-fitting and comfortable.

All of these mechanical factors—positioning, adding reinforcements, and molding—should be a part of the instinctive ability of the individual who often applies plaster-of-paris casts. It is hardly possible to think in terms of doing these things specifically at the time the cast is being applied. The practitioner must have an over-all grasp of the fundamentals in order to form a strong, stable cast.

Drying Times

The drying times of plaster can be varied tremendously by additives included by various manufacturers. Wide ranges of faster or slower drying plasters can be purchased. The average drying time is indicated in minutes on the packages; the drying time required can be selected after reading the labels. For the physician who only occasionally applies plaster casts, the selection of a moderate- to slow-drying plaster is preferable. This allows greater ease in application of the cast and longer available time for molding and positioning the cast. The practitioner who applies casts often enough to be adept in their use may want a relatively fast-drying plaster. He can handle it quite properly, and can benefit from the saving of time that the fast-drying plaster affords. The experienced practitioner will find, even with the use of ultrafast-drying plaster, that he is able to mold the cast quite efficiently; he can achieve proper position and strength strictly as a matter of experience.

The extremely fast-drying plasters are also important in treatment by corrective casts of infants and children. It is imperative that the cast dry very rapidly, since the extremity often must be held against the resistance of a struggling child. The faster the plaster dries, the more likely the position will be acceptable once drying is complete.

The fast-drying plasters are usually used in emergency rooms where it is necessary to hold reductions achieved by closed manipulation while the plaster dries. Again, fast-drying plaster makes it easier to accomplish this positioning satisfactorily.

Drying plaster can also be influenced by the temperature of the water used for wetting plaster rolls. Cold water makes all plasters slower drying; conversely, increasing the water temperature will increase the speed of drying. The addition of salt to the water, likewise, improves the drying speed, as does the addition of a small amount of powdered alum.

PADDING

The cast should be put on over some type of padding to protect the underlying tissue.

Sheet Wadding

The usual padding is a thin cotton material known as "sheet wadding." Sheet wadding has two compressed sides with a very thin filmy center. Sheets are cut in various widths to fashion rolls for application.

Sheet wadding is quite fluffy and constitutes a good padding material; however, it does not lie down well and is not as easy to apply uniformly. It does not follow the contour of the extremity well and bunches or forms ridges; even though the material is soft, it may produce ridging of the skin.

Webril

Most of the newer padding materials are of a coarser weave. They adhere better and are more evenly applied (Fig. 4-1). Newer paddings (such as one marketed by Curity—Webril) have a much greater tensile strength, but may cause circumferential constriction under the cast. If the padding is applied, however, with disruption of continuity each time that a turn is made around the extremity, the tendency for circumferential constriction is minimized. This material also has the capacity to adhere to itself, so that a very nice, smooth, even application is possible.

Other types of cast padding in use are compromises between the regular sheet wadding and Webril. The padding is much softer and is quilted to allow for a greater amount of padding. It is fashioned so that the sides are not slick; therefore, the material is easier to apply and can be made to follow the contour of the extremity better than regular sheet wadding.

Padding Over Bony Prominences

In addition to material that is wrapped around the extremity, material is used also as an additional padding over bony prominences. An example is orthopedic felt that is contoured to fit the iliac crest to help protect it while applying a body spica cast. Strips of felt may be split and contoured by stretching so that they fit nicely over the bony prominences. Foam rubber also is used for this additional padding. Foam rubber is softer than the felt, but tends to absorb odors. Occasionally, it causes hypersensitivity reactions. The newer foam plastic padding is more acceptable. This material is extremely soft and does not absorb odors as much as does foam rubber. Its use is preferable to both the felt and the foam-rubber paddings.

Padding should be applied judiciously. When a great amount of padding is interposed between the cast and the extremity, some efficiency is lost; fractures that otherwise might be stable in a cast will lose position because of the amount of play that occurs between the extremity and the cast.

Padding should be applied smoothly. Even though the cast padding material is quite soft, there is a danger of pressure phenomena if the padding is built up excessively. When the padding is applied circumferentially into a large roll, compromise in circulation may occur distal to the area of constriction. By the same token, when padding material is applied over bony prominences, care must be taken that this does not make the prominent area more exposed to pressure under the cast.

PRESSURE POINTS

When a great amount of swelling is anticipated, the minimal amount of padding should be applied, and the cast should be split so as to allow for the swelling. The padding should be applied so that it can be split easily and the swelling allowed to progress unimpeded. Again, padding should not increase

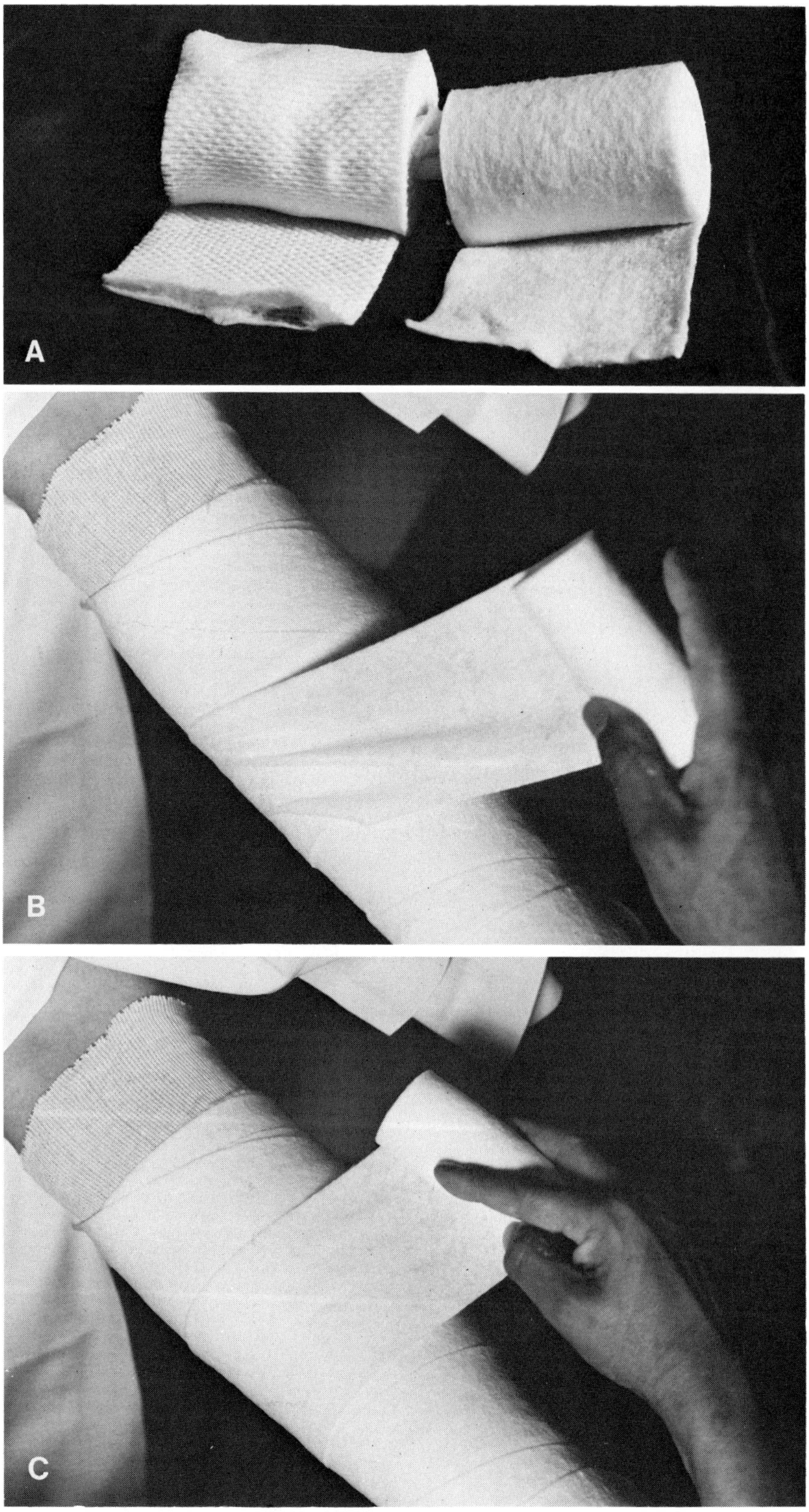

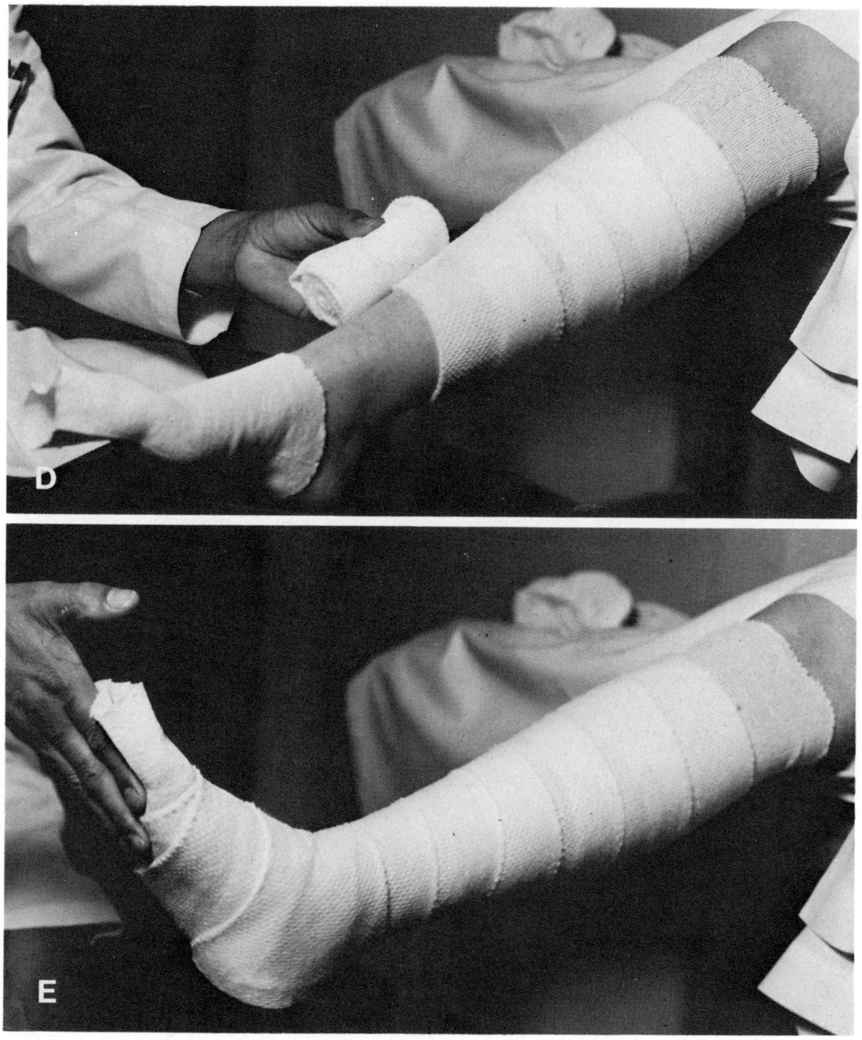

Fig. 4-1. (A) Cast padding. *(Right)* Webril has a much closer weave and is much stronger, so that stretching is not as easy. It conforms much better than the fluffier cast padding *(left)*, which does allow for more compaction when swelling occurs, is much less manageable, and much more difficult to apply smoothly. *(B and C)* Application of Webril. *(D and E)* Application of fluffy cast padding.

pressure over normal bony prominences. If a large, bulky amount of padding is applied in certain area, it forms a prominence. A pressure area will occur under the cast simply from a rolling up of padding material.

Careful application and sparing use of the padding material will allow for a much more effective cast, and at the same time will be effective in preventing the formation of pressure points. The proper molding of the cast around the bony prominences, following the normal contour of the extremity, is much more important in preventing pressure areas than is the application of great amounts of padding. (See Fig. 3-4.) If the cast is molded carefully, even with scanty padding, it is not likely to cause pressure phenomena, particularly if swelling is anticipated and the cast is split to allow for it.

Indentations

If the cast is not properly held while drying, the marks of the fingers are likely to form indentations. These dents form abnormal pressure areas on the extremity. Dents may also occur when the flexion of a joint is changed during this drying stage. This occurs, for instance, in the case of casts in which the knee is held in a certain position while the cast is applied, but during the drying stage the knee is allowed to flex further. Indentation of the cast at the flexion crease will result in a prominent pressure point within the cast.

Windowing

After the cast has hardened, if the patient complains of any pressure whatsoever, he should not be ignored. The area that causes the patient discomfort should be inspected. If it appears that a pressure area does exist, a window should be cut out over the area with a cast saw, the padding removed so that the skin can be inspected, a foam-rubber or plastic foam pad applied in this window, and the window reapplied with tape.

It is a mistake to remove an area of the cast and leave an open window without reapplying some type of pressure. If a window is left as an opening in the cast, swelling of the extremity is likely to occur through the window. There is danger of pressure areas occurring around the margins of the window. If the window is opened and the area inspected, a soft plastic foam pad inserted, and the window replaced with tape, the cause of the pressure to the skin will be eliminated. At the same time, the firm gentle pressure of the soft plastic foam pad will prevent swelling of this area through the window.

One of the typical complaints of patients with pressure areas in their casts is burning pain. Prolonged pressure even of relatively low intensity over an area of skin is interpreted by the patient as a "burning pain"; particular attention should be given to the patient with this complaint. Abnormal pressure over a relatively small area produces agonizing pain over a period of time since the pressure is continuous. Skin sensitivity is great enough to cause severe pain over these areas.

As mentioned previously, these complaints by the patients should never be ignored; the pressure areas should be inspected. It is preferable to reapply a cast rather than to continue a cast that seems to be producing multiple pressure areas. Pressure sores that develop under the cast are extremely hard to heal. They may result in indolent ulcers that require much time and treatment in an effort to effect a cure. *Pressure sores are much easier to prevent than to treat once they have occurred.*

METHOD OF APPLICATION

While there are many methods of applying casts and many variations in technique, the general principles are the same for all. The method described here is basically one that has been used effectively by the author over a period of many years. The practitioner who applies casts will develop variations of this technique, and will find new techniques that work well in his own hands.

Preparation

Preparation of the extremity begins with inspection of the skin to be certain that no rash exists and that surgical or traumatic wounds are in good condition. Casts should never, under any circumstances, be applied over an area of skin eruption; the rash will invariably become worse. Small areas, perhaps, can be covered, and then immediately exposed by windows cut with the cast saw after the cast is applied. Open wounds should also be exposed by windowing so that they can be redressed and treated.

A window can be made in the cast for inspection of surgical wounds or for removal of the sutures. Many operators prefer skin tapes for wound closures when a cast is to be applied. This obviates removal of sutures after the wound has healed. Most operators, however, feel that at least a small window should be made over the wound after a period of time has elapsed. This may be done, whether or not sutures are present, to inspect the wound for infection, marginal slough, or other wound complications.

Stockinett. The use of stockinett is advocated by many cast technicians, but it is not necessary for the application of an excellent cast. Stockinett supplies a smooth covering over the skin and allows trimming of the ends of the cast to make them more smooth (Fig. 4-2). On the other hand, if the stockinett is pulled tightly in areas of prominence, such as over the heel, the stockinett itself can act as a pressure point and can cause pressure areas to develop. Also, if care is not taken to avoid folding or wrinkling of the stockinett, particularly over flexion creases, pressure areas can result that may cause ulcerations under the cast. Many experienced cast technicians prefer to apply cast padding directly over the skin, or at the very most to use two small sections of stockinett at the two ends of the cast for trimming the cast margins, rather than for encompassing the entire extremity. When stockinett is not used it is very simple to fold over the cast padding and make a very smooth margin. One additional difficulty with the use of stockinett is that it requires additional handling of the extremity, resulting in loss of position of fresh fractures or increased pain to the patient, since the rolling on of stockinett requires some manipulation.

Padding. Following the application of the stockinett, if it is to be used, the cast padding is applied. It should be applied in transverse turns. If the newer types of padding are used, the padding should be torn often so that long lengths of circumferentially placed padding are not applied. Paddings may have a tourniquet effect if the more coarsely woven types are used; therefore, circumferentially placed padding without breaks in its continuity is to be avoided. When regular sheet wadding is used, it is difficult to secure the ends. The tearing off of a small portion of one side of the sheet wadding will expose some of the fluffy inner portion, allowing it to adhere to the rest and to lie down without unwinding. The judicious use of padding has been previously mentioned; however, it should be reiterated that the padding should follow very closely the contours of the extremity. It should not be used excessively, since this tends to decrease the effectiveness of the cast in immobilizing the extremity. If considerable swelling is anticipated, it is advisable to consider splitting the cast after application, rather than to apply excessive padding to allow for the swelling. If felt pads are to be used, they should be applied on top of the regular sheet wadding so that they will become adherent to the undersurface of

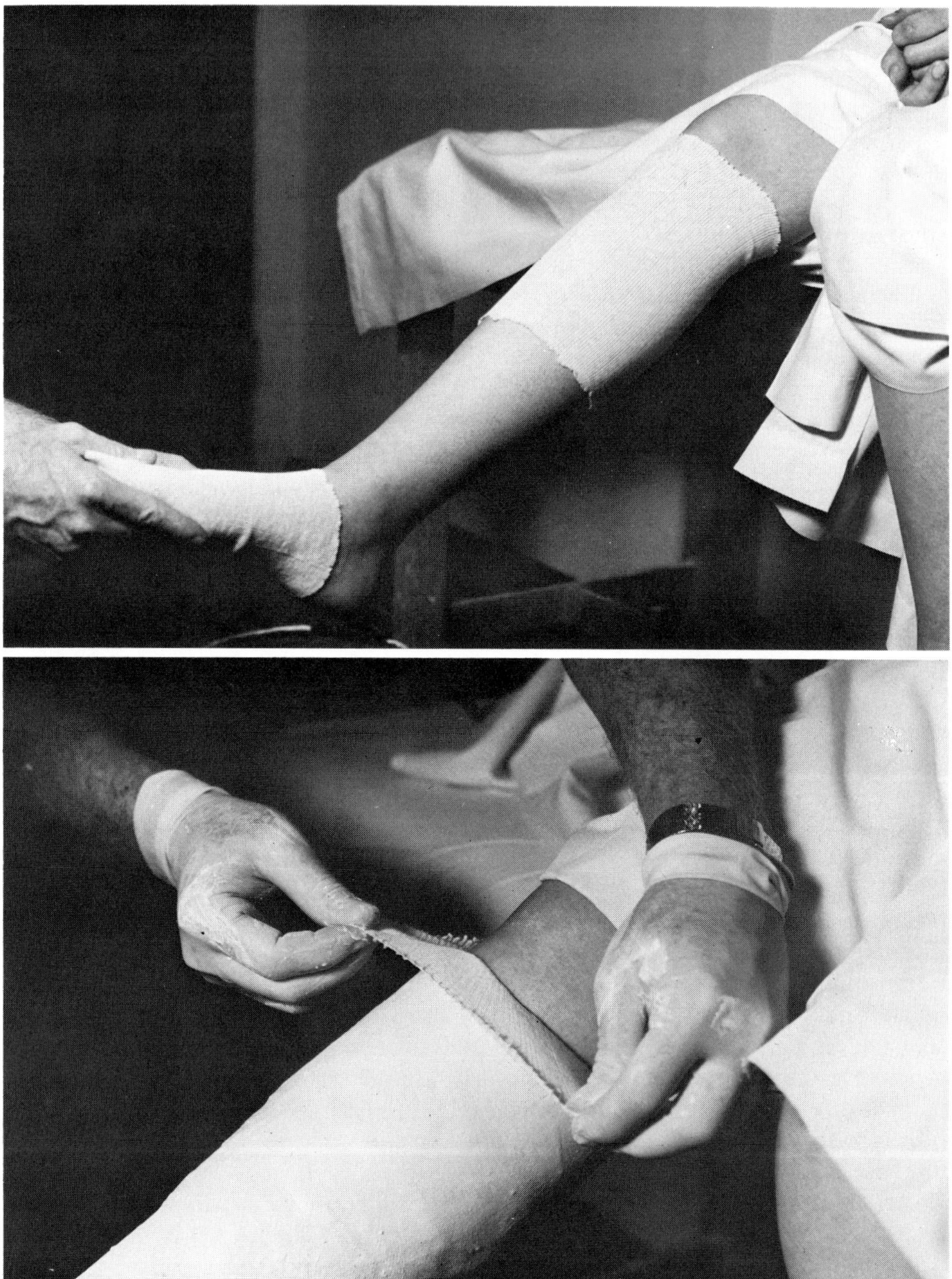

Fig. 4-2. Stockinett is shown in the application of a cast. It is not necessary to cover the entire extremity with stockinett, but segments of it at either end of the cast are valuable for aid in trimming the cast and holding the padding and plaster together. The stockinett at either end can be folded over and incorporated in the plaster while the cast is being applied.

the cast. If felt pads migrate under the cast, they will sometimes cause pressure areas.

Applying The Plaster

The plaster rolls are rolled into place to form the cast. The larger roll, rather than a smaller one, should be used. Not only is the cast smoother when larger rolls are used, but also there is less chance with the larger rolls of forming a circumferential constricted area. Attempts should be made to get by with 6-inch plaster rolls alone. Particularly in the lower extremity is it possible to use the wider plaster, even on the average size adult foot. When smaller casts are applied, such as on the hand and forearm, however, it is better to use a narrower width such as 3-inch or 4-inch plaster. The 2-inch rolls are necessary when applying small club foot casts or casts to other small areas.

Wetting. The water for immersion should be as hot as can be tolerated comfortably, since this allows faster drying. Additives to the water may be used, as have been previously described. The container should be deep enough to allow a water level that will completely cover the rolls when they stand on end. The rolls should be dropped into the water longitudinally so that they stand on end; they should be left in the water until air bubbles stop rising to the surface. This indicates that complete wetting of the plaster has occurred (Fig. 4-3). The plaster roll should be removed from the water and grasped with one end in each hand. In this position the roll can be gently squeezed and rolled to assure uniform distribution of plaster throughout the roll. At the same time, the ends can be tightly squeezed to prevent telescoping of the roll. The rolls should never be wrung out, as in wringing out a towel. This will result in loss of much of the incorporated plaster by forcing it out in the squeezing process. This also removes an excessive amount of water so that the plaster is difficult to apply and dries during the rolling process. Leaving a large amount of liquid plaster within the roll insures that the plaster will become incorporated into the cast as a solid homogeneous unit. A better structured cast will result if there is a longer period of time available for molding the cast to the extremity.

Rolling. The plaster should be rolled onto the extremity in a transverse manner. Care should be taken to avoid pulling the crinoline bandage too tightly; this will result in circumferential pressure areas inside the cast. As the

(Text continued on page 78.)

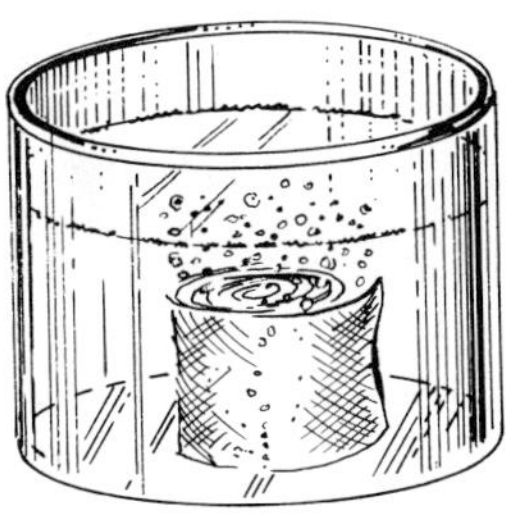

Fig. 4-3. The plaster roll is dipped into a container of water that contains more than enough to cover the roll standing on its end. The longitudinal position of the roll is much better than allowing it lie flat in the basin, since this allows for better incorporation of water into the roll. The roll is left in this position until all bubbles disappear.

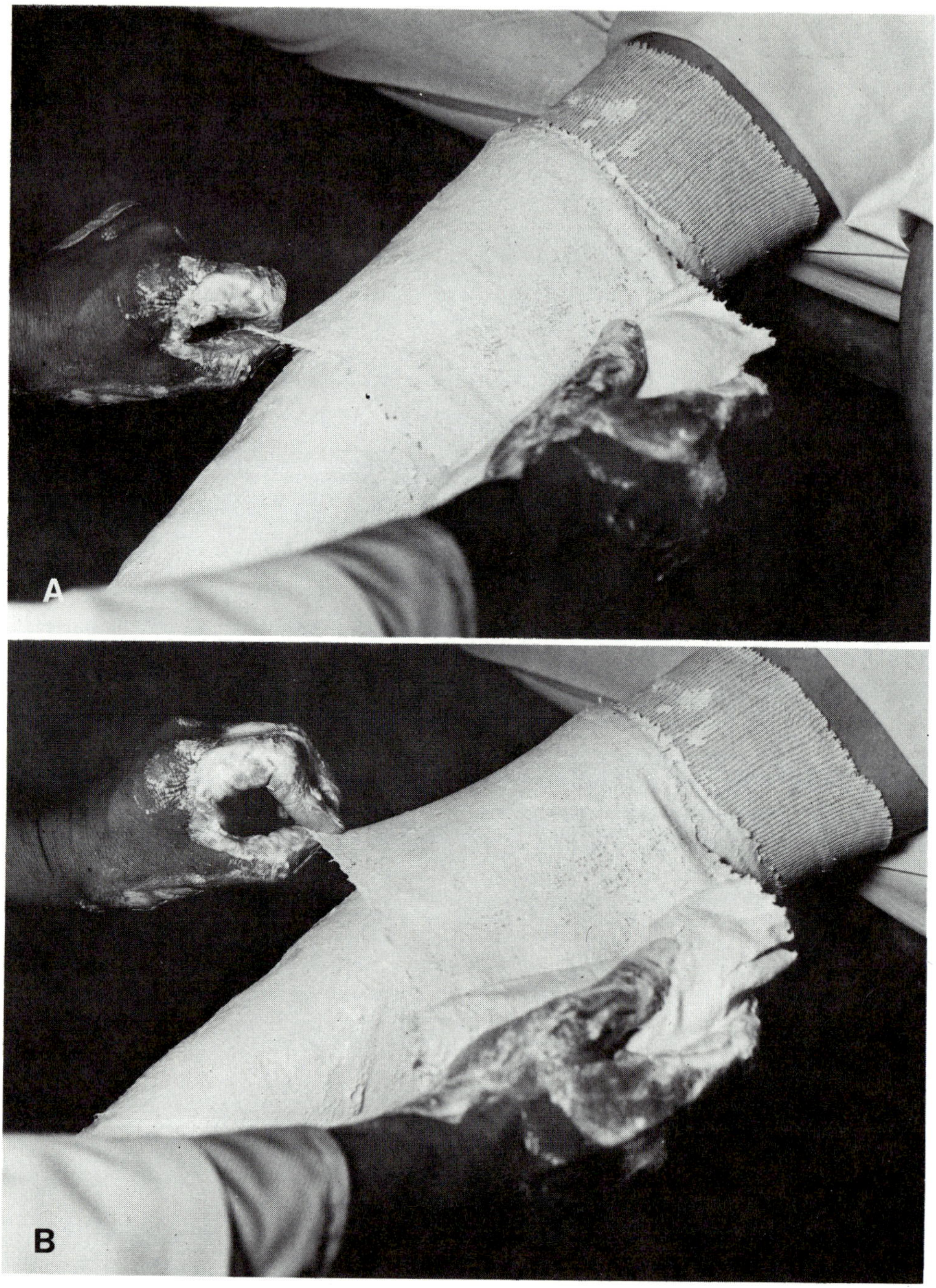

Fig. 4-4. (A) When rolling plaster, the plaster should be held so that the individual turns are approximately transverse. This leaves the proximal portion of the turn much tighter than the distal portion, when the plaster is being applied to an area with decreasing circumference. *(B)* The left hand catches the loose portion of the free margin distally and creates a fold, so that the tightness of the distal margin of the roll is as tight as the proximal. This fold can then be covered as the plaster is advanced by subsequent turns down the leg. *(Legend continued on opposite page.)*

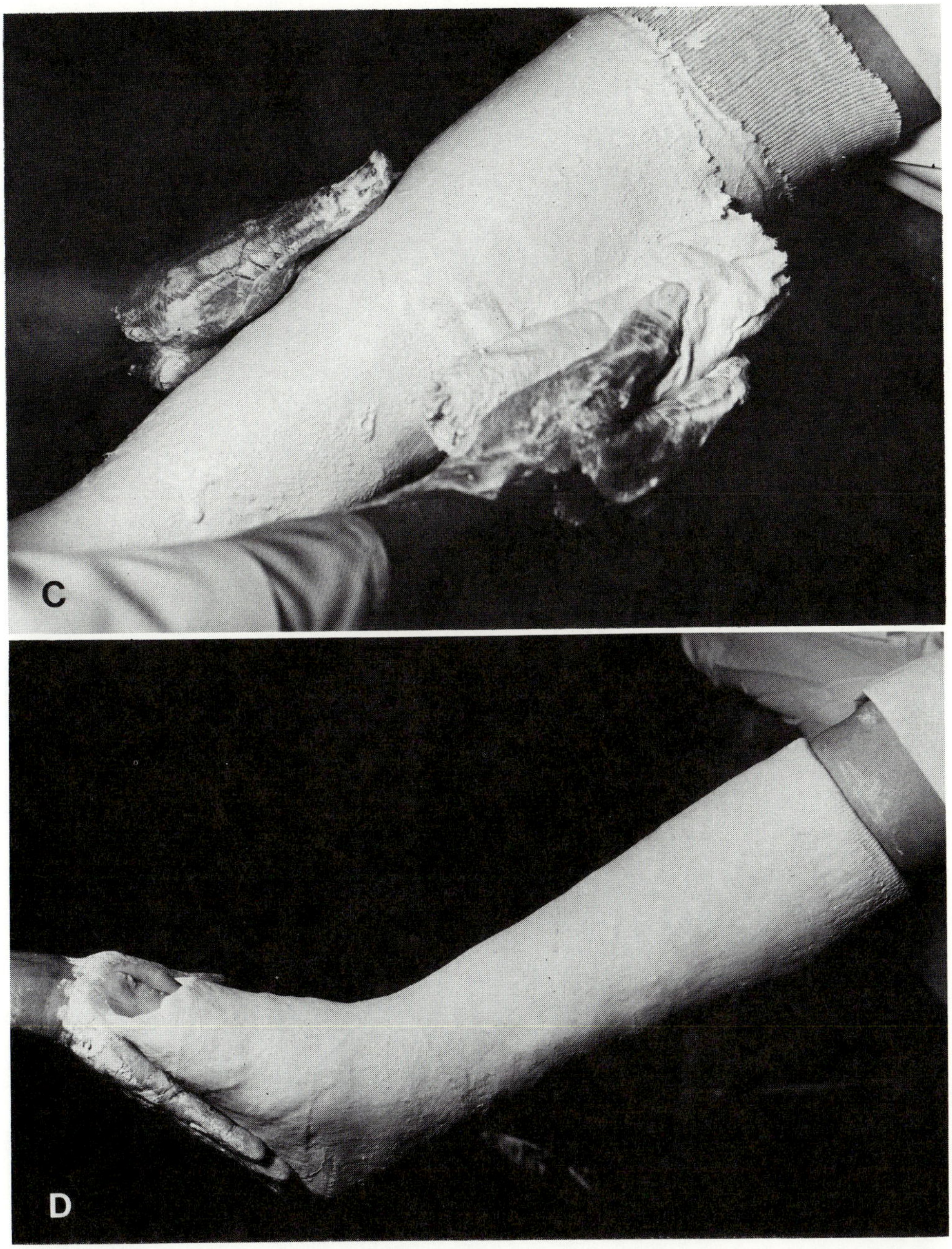

Fig. 4-4, continued. (C) Molding the plaster by massage as turns are made. *(D)* The finished cast.

contour of the extremity changes, the plaster should be rolled still in a transverse manner. The smaller area of the extremity can be fitted by pulling out the slack in the bandage as it is wound, creating a tuck that can be folded over and laid smoothly against the extremity (Fig. 4-4). This will allow for a very neat application of the plaster bandage. It will follow the contour with optimal molding to the shape of the extremity. Each successive turn of the bandage should overlap the preceding layer by about one half of its width, so that no two rolls are exactly lying over each other. As the bandage is passed around a joint, such as a flexed knee or an ankle held at 90 degrees, a figure-of-eight pattern can be used to allow for equal distribution of the plaster. Again, the successive roll should not exactly overlap the previous one, but should overlap enough so that there is a continuity of the rolls without excessive thickness in a single area. If the plaster is rolled on with the right hand, the tucks can be taken with the left hand, and the left hand can be further used to smooth out the plaster as it is applied.

Molding. It is very important to massage continuously the layers of plaster as they are applied so that the plaster is uniformly distributed through the crinoline network to form a homogeneous mass. The massage should be done with the palmar surfaces of the hands and fingers, and should be done in such a manner as to gently force the plaster over the various contours of the extremity (Fig.4-5). If careful molding is done, the cast does not need to be thick to be

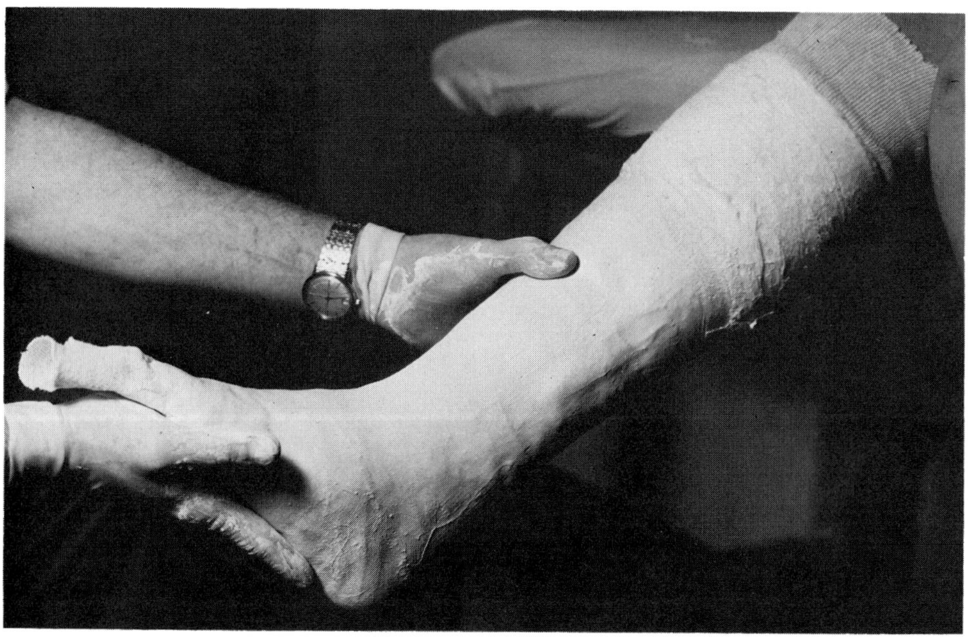

Fig. 4-5. While the cast is being applied, it is extremely important to massage the contour of the cast, so that the pliable plaster is made to closely follow the contours of the extremity. As the plaster dries, the molding process is continued until the plaster has "set." Rubbing over bony prominences and irregular contours is done with both hands simultaneously, and is done vigorously enough so that the plaster conforms closely to the contour of the extremity.

strong and effective. On the contrary, a well molded, thinly padded, lightweight cast is more effective. If the cast is not massaged and molded so that a homogenous mass is created, lamination may occur, with subsequent loss of strength and destruction of the stability of the cast. The plaster should never be twisted upon itself when rolling. This allows for a pressure area to develop and results in ridging of the cast. Reverses are sometimes necessary over particularly prominent areas such as the heel, but these can be applied without difficulty by passing the roll back and forth over the palm of the hand and laying out a small pad of plaster several layers thick before applying it to the area.

Reinforcing. Straight plaster splints are produced by commercial manufacturers in widths varying from 3 to 6 inches. These splints also vary in length, but can be adjusted to any size desired for a particular area. When additional strength of a cast is needed, these plaster splints form the ideal way to apply this extra strength. They can be applied in a longitudinal manner, as contrasted with the transverse manner in which the plaster-of-paris bandages are applied from rolls. Additional strength around joints such as the knee, which is held in the flexed position for casting, must be provided to prevent breaking of the cast. The simplest and most efficient way to supply this additional strength is by incorporating additional longitudinal plaster splints in the circular bandage as it is applied.

Preventing Telescoping. Occasionally, the center of the roll will slip out of the roll in a phenomenon known as "telescoping." When this occurs to the extent that the central portion of the roll becomes completely displaced from the remainder, it is necessary to completely discard the remainder of the roll and start with a fresh one. The tendency to telescope can be greatly diminished by squeezing a small portion of the margin of each end of the wet plaster roll. This binds the ends together and prevents the slipping out of the central portion of the roll. Likewise, telescoping can be handled better when it first begins to occur by merely using the thumb or finger to press the telescoping center of the bandage back into its normal relationship, before it slips completely out of the roll. Some types of plaster tend to telescope more easily than others; some manufacturers provide a small cardboard or plastic core for the roll, which tends to diminish tremendously the possibility of telescoping.

Trimming. The cast should always be applied somewhat longer than is needed. Once the plaster has set and dried, the margins can be trimmed back to the appropriate position. It is seldom possible to apply the cast directly up to the precise level that one desires while holding it on. If the cast is made slightly longer than is desired, a single-edged razor blade or a cast knife can be used to trim the cast carefully, cutting it at the desired level after the cast has dried. Once the cast has dried and has been trimmed, a somewhat thicker margin can be created at the end of the cast, which helps prevent breakdown of the cast margins. After trimming of the plaster has been accomplished, the padding or stockinett can be folded over the top and bottom of the cast and secured with an additional roll of plaster. This gives a very soft margin to the cast, which is not only more pleasing in appearance but also more comfortable to wear.

In the case of the toe portion of a boot cast, many operators prefer to trim the cast in such a manner as to leave a platform on which the toes can rest. This is necessary if the foot has a tendency to develop a toe-drop or flexion contractures of toes; where normal toes exist, the platform is not particularly neces-

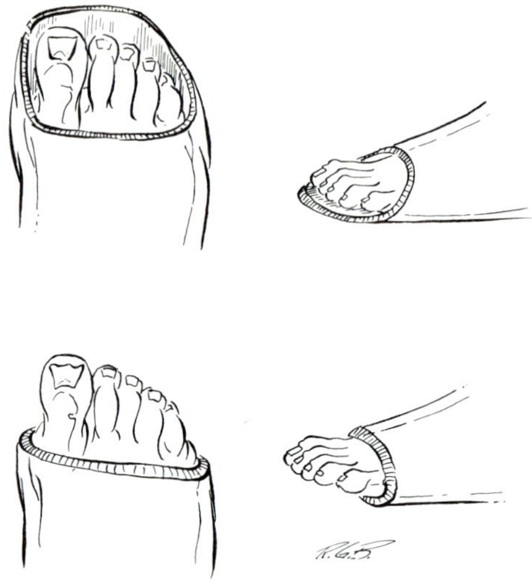

Fig. 4-6. Trimming of the cast is done after the plaster application and setting has been completed. The set plaster is trimmed while still damp, using a sharp blade. If stockinett has been used prior to the cast application, it can be folded over the cast padding and plaster margins and sealed with an additional strip of plaster. In the case of a lower extremity cast, a platform can be left to support the toes and prevent toe-drop formation. Some practitioners favor leaving the toes completely exposed without a platform underneath, so that vigorous exercise of the toes can be accomplished.

sary. The cast should be extended out past the metatarsal heads, in any event, to give maximum support to the foot (Fig. 4-6). If the platform is desired, the cast should be extended out past the end of the toes and the upper portion trimmed back with a cast knife to expose the toes. Following the application of a cast, all toes or fingers should be left exposed. In no event should a cast extend out past the toes for any length of time; this will result in maceration of the web space between the toes and development of ulcerations and infection.

The trimming of the cast, as mentioned, can be done with a straight-edged razor blade, a regular cast knife, or a scalpel. The cast knife that is made for trimming the casts tends to become dull. Since its blade is retained for long periods of time, frequent sharpening with a file is necessary to keep it sharp enough to cut the plaster effectively. For this reason, many operators prefer the use of the single-edge razor blade or a scalpel that has a disposable blade; a new one is provided for each case.

Splitting. When considerable swelling is anticipated, the cast should be split. This is particularly true for lower extremity casts. Splitting should be done as soon as the cast is applied. It is much easier to do at this time and much more convenient than waiting until the swelling has occurred, necessitating immediate splitting of the cast at inconvenient hours. Splitting may be done with the cast knife or blade if it is done soon after the cast has dried. Otherwise, it is necessary to use the cast saw to remove a small strip of the plaster. It is better to remove a strip of plaster 1 or 2 cm. in width, than to cut a single slit in the cast to allow for the anticipated swelling. (See Fig. 3-5). The removal of the strip of cast does not seriously compromise the strength or stability of the cast but does make it easier to spread the cast if it becomes necessary when swelling occurs. Cutting of a strip from the cast also allows for inspection or cutting of the underlying padding if the swelling becomes severe. If a strip has been cut, it is much simpler to introduce bandage scissors under the padding and to cut it the entire length of the split. It is mandatory that this padding be cut when swelling has become severe; the padding may result in circumferential constriction with a tourniquet effect that further compromises circulation to the distal portion of the extremity.

SPICA CAST

When it becomes necessary to include the hip or the shoulder with an immobilized extremity held in a plaster cast, a so-called spica cast is used. This term implies the inclusion of the entire upper or lower extremity with the extension of the cast across the shoulder or hip joint onto the body.

Hip Spica

Typically, the hip spica extends from the tip of the toes to the lower portion of the thoracic cage proximally on the involved side (Fig. 4-7). Whether or not all or a portion of the opposite leg is included depends upon the judgment of the physician and the condition to be treated. If completely secure fixation of the pelvis is desired, it becomes obvious that the contralateral hip must be immobilized. Without inclusion of the opposite hip and at least a portion of the opposite extremity, the pelvis will display a considerable range of motion in both the lateral and the sagittal plane. Unless the opposite extremity is involved in some way, it is usually not necessary to extend the cast below the knee of the uninvolved side. The short side of the cast should be terminated high enough that complete motion of the uninvolved knee can be achieved by the patient. Care must be taken that the cast is trimmed posteriorly high enough to allow motion without impingement of the soft tissue on the cast margin. Care also must be taken that the margin is smooth and rounded to prevent irritation of the skin. If it is not necessary to include the other extremity, the cast can be trimmed so that the long-leg cast on the involved side is merely extended to include a pelvic, or, if somewhat higher, a torso band. This cast is referred to as a single spica as contrasted to a "one and one-half" or a "double spica" when part or all of the other extremity is included.

Stabilizing. In the one-and-one-half and the double spicas, structural stability is not great enough to withstand breakage across the hip joint areas unless a bar of plaster is placed across the interval between the legs to stabilize the cast, transforming an unstable "V" into a more stable triangle. Many operators prefer to cut a small piece of wood, approximately 2 or 3 cm. in cross-sectional diameter, to appropriate length and, after wrapping it in wet plaster bandages, apply it to the legs of the cast with additional plaster. Many have found it more convenient to provide this stabilizing strut by attaching a plaster "twist" in the location between the legs. This technique involves the use of plaster splints (approximately 10 thicknesses) in lengths slightly longer than the distance to be traversed. These 5-inch or 6-inch splints can then be twisted so that a roll or "rod" of plaster is developed with two free flaps on either end. These loose flaps can then be applied to both the front and back side of either leg. They are

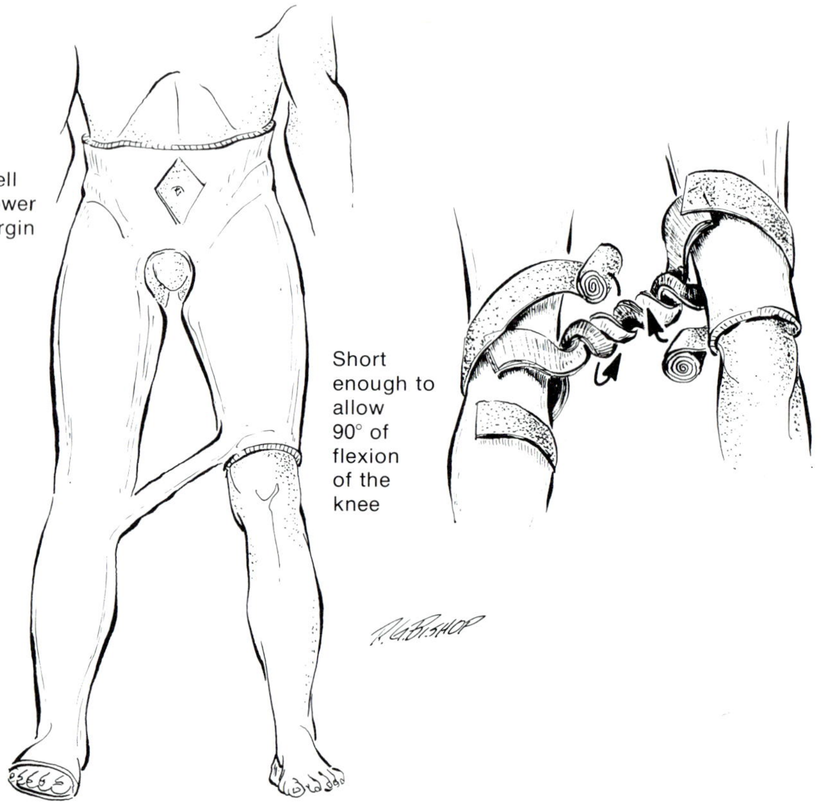

Fig. 4-7. A one-and-one-half spica cast, extending from the lower rib margin to the tips of the toes on the involved side, and to the knee on the opposite side. Generally, the hip is held in slight abduction in order to separate the legs enough to allow for peroneal care. A support is necessary between the short segment and the major segment of the cast. This is fashioned by using a "twist" (*right*). Plaster splints are wound together, leaving two ends free at either end of the twist. These are then wrapped around the legs of the cast on either side, and, using roll plaster, they are secured to the legs of the cast. The twist is covered with multiple layers of plaster from the roll, so that a very smooth, sturdy, well-incorporated support is manufactured.

attached by additional rolls of plaster bandage which are not only rolled around the legs to attach the flaps, but also are rolled circumferentially around the plaster rod to keep it round and to keep the layers of splints closely squeezed together. The rod is quite limp when first applied, but with a short time of rubbing and wrapping with additional rolls of bandage, it becomes quite rigid and creates a very satisfactory stabilizing rod (Fig. 4-7, *right*).

After the cast has been applied, it must be trimmed anteriorly in the pubic area, as well as on either side, and posteriorly to a point above the cleft between the buttocks so that personal hygiene can be accomplished. The margins on either side should occur down on the upper thigh a short distance below—but not within—the inguinal crease. The margins should be smooth; more comfort can be achieved if the margins are broken back 1 cm. to make them softer, before the plaster dries completely. After the cast is dry (24 to 48 hours) a diamond-shaped abdominal window may be cut. It should not be large, since it may weaken the cast, and it should be located over the epigastrium to allow for fullness after eating. The same general precautions should be observed in spica casts as in all casts, concerning padding, pressure points, and the like.

The Cast Syndrome. In describing the hip spica cast, a word should be included concerning the "cast syndrome." It has long been recognized that the application of a cast that covers the abdomen may result in severe ileus. Whether this is due to immobility or to some autonomic alteration is a matter of some conjecture. The fact remains, however, that this can often be a very distressing situation, with the ileus being severe enough to compromise respiration by pressing on the diaphragm. These patients are often frightened to a panic stage by the thought that they cannot breathe. The symptoms often become so distressing that the anterior aspect of the abdominal segment of the cast must be split and spread to make more room. These patients are usually quite anxious to begin with; most practitioners believe that the acuteness of the syndrome is accentuated markedly by air swallowing. Decompression with a nasogastric tube is necessary for a day or so until the abdomen has become entirely flat. The cast then can be safely repaired across the abdomen without problems. As a general rule, it is better to keep these patients on only liquids by mouth for the first 24 to 48 hours following spica cast application, to minimize the cases where this severe abdominal distention occurs. Even when no distention occurs, elimination by the intestinal tract may be very sluggish; careful attention should be given to use of enemas, laxatives, or stool softeners, as indicated.

Care of the patient in a spica cast follows routine measures. Personal hygiene is very important. If this is observed carefully, usually no real problems are encountered. The patient can be turned and moved about without restriction, as long as he remains horizontal. It is even permissible to allow movement on a stretcher, as desired, unless some specific contraindication exists. Moving the patient about from room to room and even out of doors when weather permits is very important to prevent the boredom that accompanies the detention of an otherwise healthy individual in a single room. A simple homemade stretcher is adequate, as long as it is sturdy enough to prevent dropping. Such a stretcher can even be made from an old panel door, or perhaps borrowed from a local ambulance company. Patients who have only a single spica may occasionally be allowed up on crutches. In some instances, single spica casts may be applied with the foot remaining free so that a shoe and sock can be worn for partial weightbearing. These privileges should be allowed only at the discretion and upon the orders of the attending physician.

Shoulder Spica Casts

Shoulder spica casts have few of the implications of hip spica casts because the patient is usually ambulatory and the abdomen is not completely covered. The shoulder cast is only applied on one side, and the other arm is left entirely free. The cast generally extends from the proximal flexion crease of the palm, across the wrist with approximately 45 degrees of flexion, and then up onto the forearm and arm, with the position of the elbow being dictated by the condition being treated. From here, the cast extends up over the shoulder onto the thorax with the shoulder position being dictated by the condition being

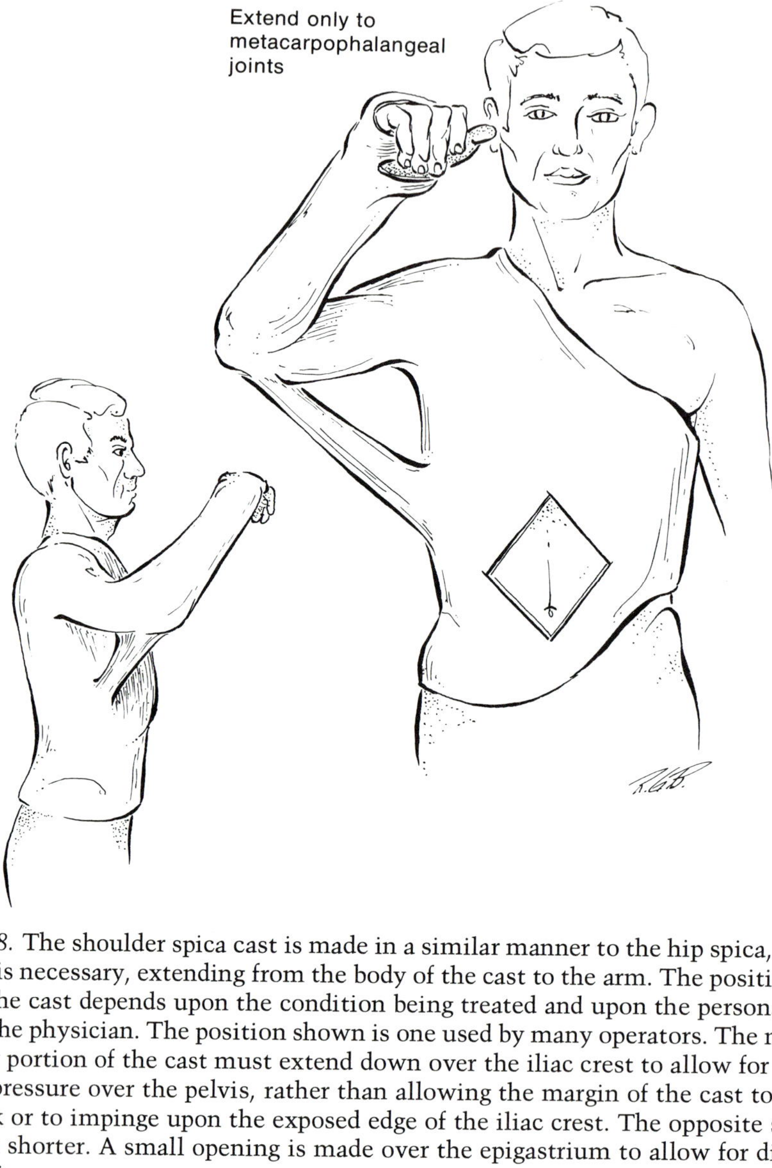

Fig. 4-8. The shoulder spica cast is made in a similar manner to the hip spica, in that a support is necessary, extending from the body of the cast to the arm. The position of the arm in the cast depends upon the condition being treated and upon the personal preference of the physician. The position shown is one used by many operators. The margin of the body portion of the cast must extend down over the iliac crest to allow for transference of pressure over the pelvis, rather than allowing the margin of the cast to cut into the flank or to impinge upon the exposed edge of the iliac crest. The opposite side may be much shorter. A small opening is made over the epigastrium to allow for distention after eating.

treated. (A position of approximately 45 degrees glenohumeral abduction is usually most comfortable.) The cast is then extended onto the thorax and either ended at the lower rib margins, or, if greater stability is desired, extended down to include the iliac crests. It is cut diagonally across the chest both anteriorly and posteriorly and crossed under the opposite arm several centimeters below the axilla. If extension to the iliac crests is necessary, the diamond-shaped abdominal window over the epigastrium should be made. The supporting rod made of a wooden strut or plaster "twist" should extend from the region of the elbow to the distal margin of the body portion (Fig. 4-8). The medial epicondyle (and occasionally the adjacent ulnar nerve) is often very prone to pressure since it is so prominent and since the arm must lie on its medial side. Great care must be taken to protect this area. If necessary, a window can be removed after the cast dries to expose the epicondyle and allow for inclusion of a polyfoam pad over the area. Elimination and gastrointestinal complications are rare in shoulder spica casts, as contrasted to their rather frequent occurrence in hip spicas. Instructions should be given for frequent active exercise of the exposed fingers and thumb to prevent stiffness.

WALKING CASTS

It occasionally is permissible to allow weightbearing in a cast, particularly when a short-leg cast is used. Some type of appliance must be applied to the cast to allow for this weightbearing. Three different appliances are commonly used.

Walking Irons

Walking irons were described by Boehler many years ago. They consist of a metallic U-shaped apparatus which is bent so that the bend of the "U" is flattened out and covered with a rubber pad to allow for weightbearing (Fig. 4-9*A*). The two uprights of the "U" are attached to the sides of the casts with plaster, actually being incorporated into the plaster as the cast is applied. The upper portion of the upright has a "T" extension to allow for better stability, particularly to prevent proximal migration when weight is applied to the bottom of the walking iron. These irons have the advantage of distributing weight up into the sides of the cast rather than directly into a small area at the bottom of the cast. They have the disadvantage of being somewhat more difficult to apply, requiring a somewhat thicker cast with a greater weight. Taking roentgenograms through the cast is much more difficult since the irons are metallic.

Walking Heel

The most common appliance used today probably is the so-called walking heel. There are a myriad of designs supplied by commercial supply houses, all of which have certain features intended to give a better gait, better stability, and to prevent the walking heel from breaking loose from the cast with weightbearing (Fig. 4-9*B*). Most of these are essentially the same from a practical standpoint; all work about as well as the others. They are applied on the plantar surface of the cast. Care should be taken that they are applied far enough posteriorly to engage the weightbearing line of the foot. If they are applied too far anteriorly, breaking of the cast through the ankle is much more likely to occur. These heels may be applied after the cast is dry by adding additional plaster to hold them on. In many instances, they are applied at the time of the original cast application. Since there is a tremendous amount of pressure applied on these heels through the base of the cast, an additional several layers of plaster in the form of splints should be applied to the sole of the cast to give additional support for the heel. Even when this is done, however, the problem occurs fairly often of softening of the cast with punching of the heel up through the sole of the cast into the foot. Likewise, the heel may

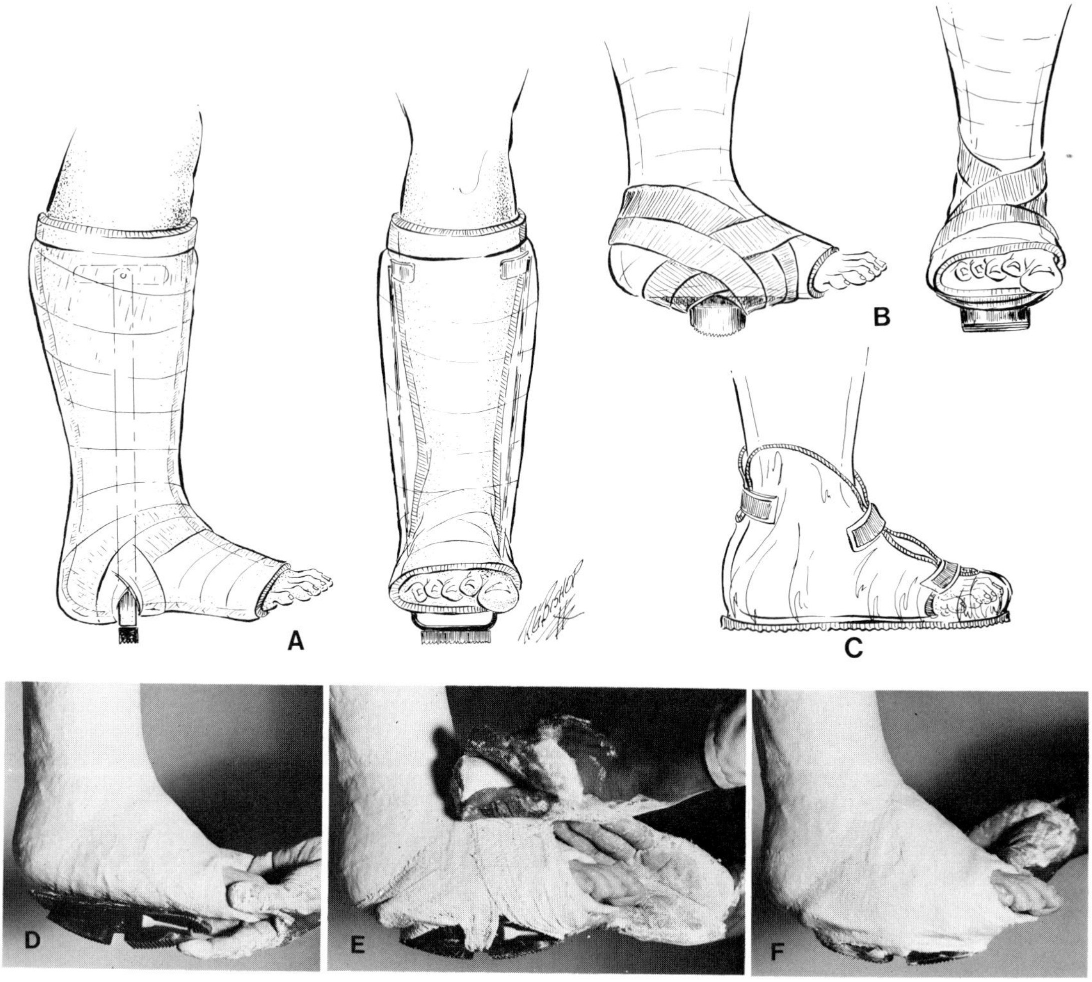

Fig. 4-9. Walking appliances. *(A)* A walking iron, which is applied with plaster extending up the side of the cast. It provides a small rubber walking surface. *(B)* A cast heel, which is applied in the central part of the foot. It is, likewise, attached to the cast with plaster, and represents a permanent portion of the cast on which weight can be borne. *(C)* A cast boot, which is applied externally to the cast to offer protection to the cast and some cushioning for weightbearing. *(D,E,F)* Application of a walking heel.

become loose with time and use and may require replacement. The most common cause of loosening of the heel, or migration of the heel up into the sole of the foot, is getting the cast wet when walking during rainy weather or through grass with dew on it. Of course, when the small area of the heel is used for the transference of the entire body weight, the amount of pressure applied to the cast is tremendous. It is not surprising that many difficulties occur with detachment of the heel. If the heel is applied properly during application of the cast, and if sufficient plaster reinforcement is applied to the cast under the heel, the result will be a satisfactory walking cast.

The patient should be requested to wear a higher heel on the contralateral foot to balance out the weightbearing level, since the walking heel does add some additional height. If the opposite shoe is built up, or if a shoe with a heel is worn to equalize the leg lengths, the patient should be able to walk reasonably well.

Cast Boot

The third method for supplying a walking cast is the so-called cast boot. This appliance is made with a sole of heavy composition material and a soft inner pad that can be applied to the foot portion of the cast with either straps or strings (Fig. 4-9*C*). The patient may walk directly on the bottom of the cast without damaging it. These boots have certain advantages: they only minimally elevate the foot, they can be attached and removed as desired, they protect the cast, particularly during rainy weather, and they can be removed at night, eliminating the weight and bulk of the other types during sleep. They have the disadvantage that they do require actual weightbearing on the foot of the cast which results in some distinct softening of the cast. If the cast has been properly reinforced, anticipating the wearing of a cast boot, this is not a serious problem.

CAST BRACING

One of the newer concepts in the treatment of fractures, particularly those of the lower extremity, concerns the use of cast bracing. Beginning with the observation of Ernst Dehne in the early 1960's, later popularized by Vert Mooney and others, the gradual development of the concept of ambulatory care of lower extremity fractures has progressed to the point where it is now a universally accepted and approved method of treatment. From the use of cast bracing in the treatment of fractures of the distal femur, as first described by Mooney, the concept has spread to the point where cast bracing is used not only with hinged casts at the knee, but also with hinges applied at the hip, elbow, wrist, and ankle. While the use of the hinged cast in joints other than the knee is still only an occasional occurrence, the hinged cast with early weightbearing in treatment of fractures of the distal femur and upper tibia is becoming a very widely used and accepted form of treatment.

In the case of other joints, the hinged cast is used basically to promote early motion in the joint and prevent joint stiffness. In the case of distal femur and upper tibial fractures, the purpose is not only to maintain motion at the knee but also to allow early ambulation with partial weightbearing on the fracture itself. The basic concept of the cast brace is that immobilization is unphysiologic while mobilization is always physiologic. Not only is the healing of the fracture promoted by the added stimulus of pressure to the fracture site, but also the ability to mobilize muscles improves circulation to the part by the massaging effect of muscles on the incorporated vessels. Motion also results in the mobilization of edema fluid that otherwise would be allowed to collect in the capsules and ligamentous structures of joints, resulting in temporary or perhaps permanent loss of function. The cast brace, then, offers the physiologic solution to many of the problems related to long continuous immobilization, either in traction or in plaster. While the basic concept of hinged cast application is essentially the same for most joints, its specific use in lower extremity fractures has developed into a technique that should be followed as closely as possible.

Method of Application (Fig. 4-10)

The cast brace is applied after the acute pain from surgical correction has subsided. During the early acute stages, the pain is great enough that the cast cannot be satisfactorily applied. As a rule, during the early stages, immobilization in a Robert-Jones dressing or other type of plaster cast is done until the acute inflammatory reaction has subsided.

The usual cast brace is applied over a Spandex cast sock. This elastic stockinett has several very desirable features which make its use almost imperative in the well-applied cast brace. By virtue of its elasticity, it creates a gentle compression force of up to 30 mm. of mercury. It follows very gently the exact contour of the extremity so that no wrinkles are allowed to occur. Further, it encompasses the tissue left exposed at the hinged area between the upper and lower segments of the cast, so that undue swelling in this unprotected segment is not likely to occur. Only a minimal amount of cast padding is necessary on top of the Spandex under the cast portions of the brace.

The cast is applied in two segments—one for the thigh and one for the leg—extending from the tibial tubercle down to the metatarsal head area, with the ankle in neutral position. The thigh portion of the cast is best applied over a molded plastic quadrilateral shell which fits the upper thigh and allows for the shaping of the musculature into the desired quadrilateral form. The upper edge is rounded for some ischial impingement, though the cast is made specifically for weightbearing by tightness on the thigh rather than for ischial weightbearing. The adjustable quadrilateral plastic shell is available commercially in different sizes to fit most any extremity. Some operators prefer to apply a single long-leg cast and cut out the knee portion. However, most have found it more practical to apply the two segments separately, with the knee area left open, so that a better fit is achieved at the margins of the cast. Once the two segments have been applied, the cast hinges are arranged on either side and are held by a jig so that the joints are maintained exactly in a parallel position. If the hinges are not held completely parallel to one another, a blocking motion will occur, limiting flexion. The jig is inserted into the appropriate part of each hinge and is held in a position so that the longitudinal axis of the hinge lies somewhat posterior to the midsagittal plane. In this position, the plane of flexion is more nearly that of the normal knee joint. While being held in this position, the two ends of the hinges are incorporated in plaster and held securely to the two segments that have already been applied and allowed to set. Most hinges have a drop-lock knee apparatus which is left fixed in full extension until complete drying of the cast has occurred. Should minor alterations be necessary once the hinges have been applied, bending irons can be used to correct any variation of position that is necessary. Once the entire cast has been allowed to dry, the Allen screw taps used to hold the drop-locks in place can be loosened and the locks can be slipped up and down as flexion is desired. The top of the lower segment of the cast must be carefully trimmed, particularly posteriorly, so that flexion is not blocked by impingement of soft tissue between the two ends of the cast segments. If immediate weightbearing is to be allowed, either a walking heel or a cast boot may be used for that purpose. For correction of angulation occurring in the fracture site or for variations required in the position of the hinges, wedging of the cast or bending of the hinges may be done, as indicated. *(Text continued on page 95.)*

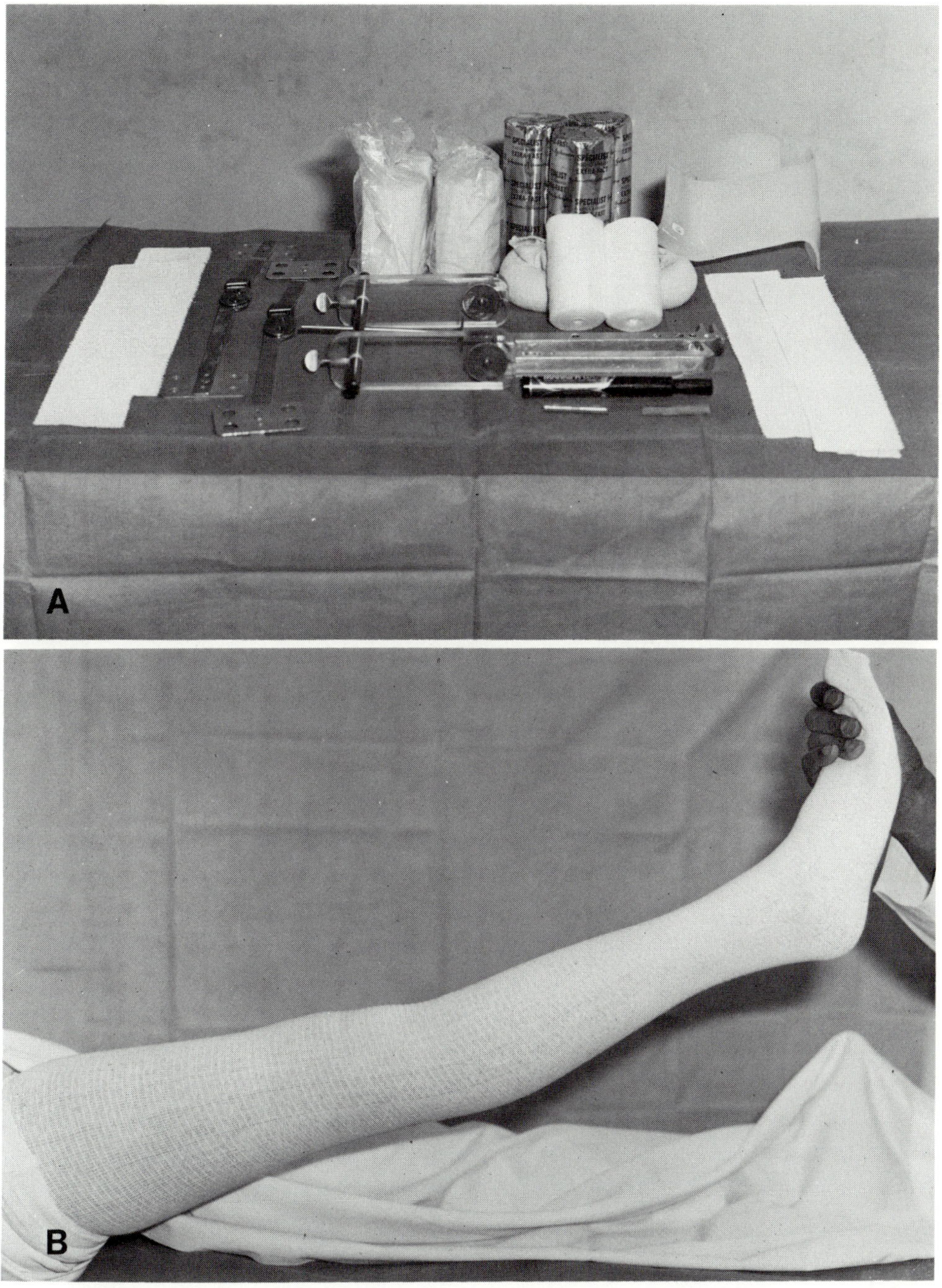

Fig. 4-10. (A) The equipment and supplies necessary for the application of a hinged cast. This includes the hinges, the guide for application of the hinges, the cast benders, and the marking tool. *(B)* The application of Spandex stockinett, which has an elastic quality that allows for compression of the extremity. *(Legend continued on overleaf.)*

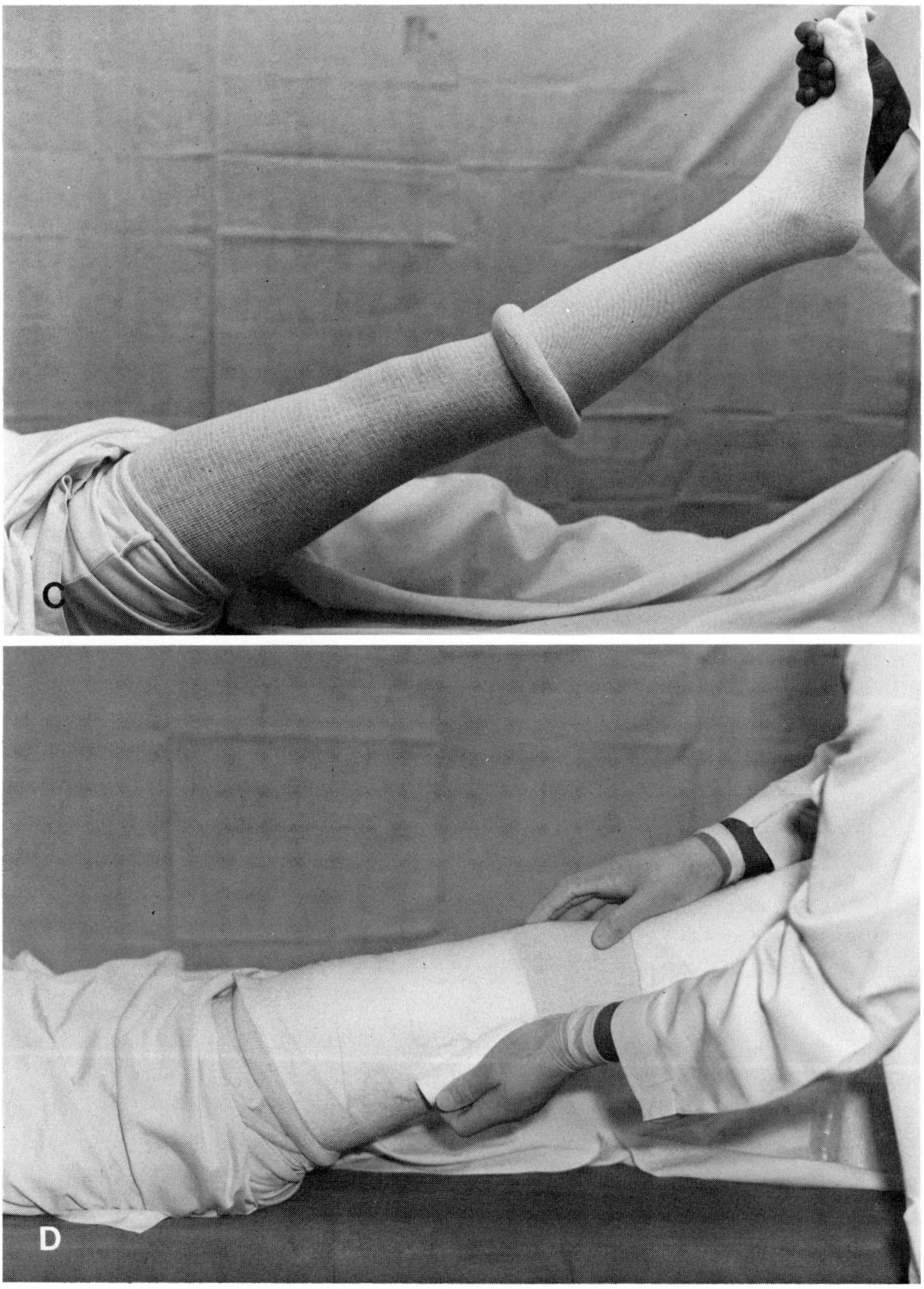

Fig. 4-10, continued. (C) The application of a second layer of regular stockinett for additional padding and binding of the margins of the two segments of the cast. *(D)* The application of cast padding over the second layer of stockinett. *(Legend continued on opposite page.)*

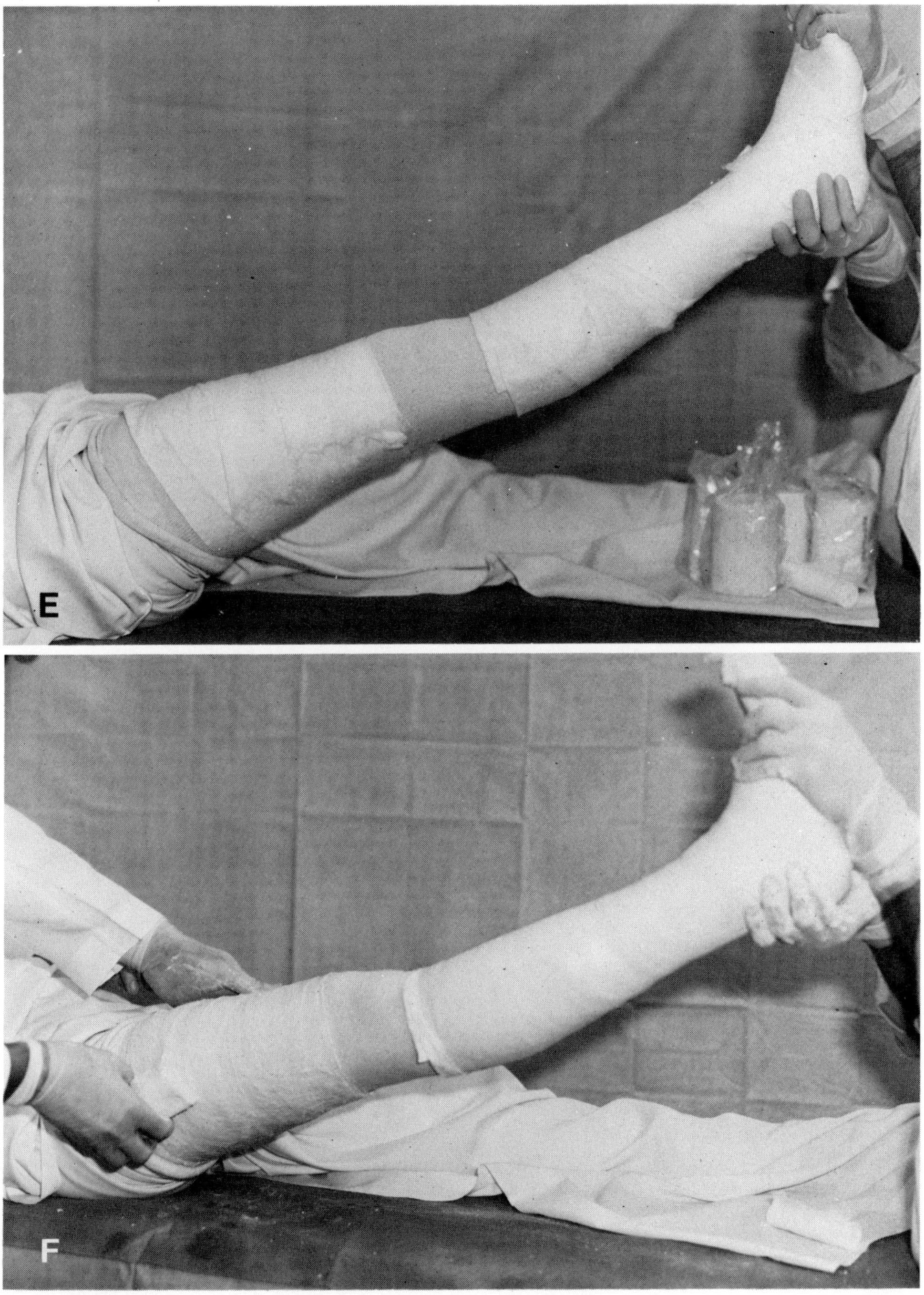

Fig. 4-10, continued. (E) The two segments of cast padding have been applied, leaving the central portion around the knee without padding, since no plaster will be used in this area. *(F)* Application of the two segments of plaster. The proximal portion is applied over a plastic cylinder, which is used to create the proximal portion of the cast with a quadrilateral weightbearing feature. *(Legend continued on overleaf.)*

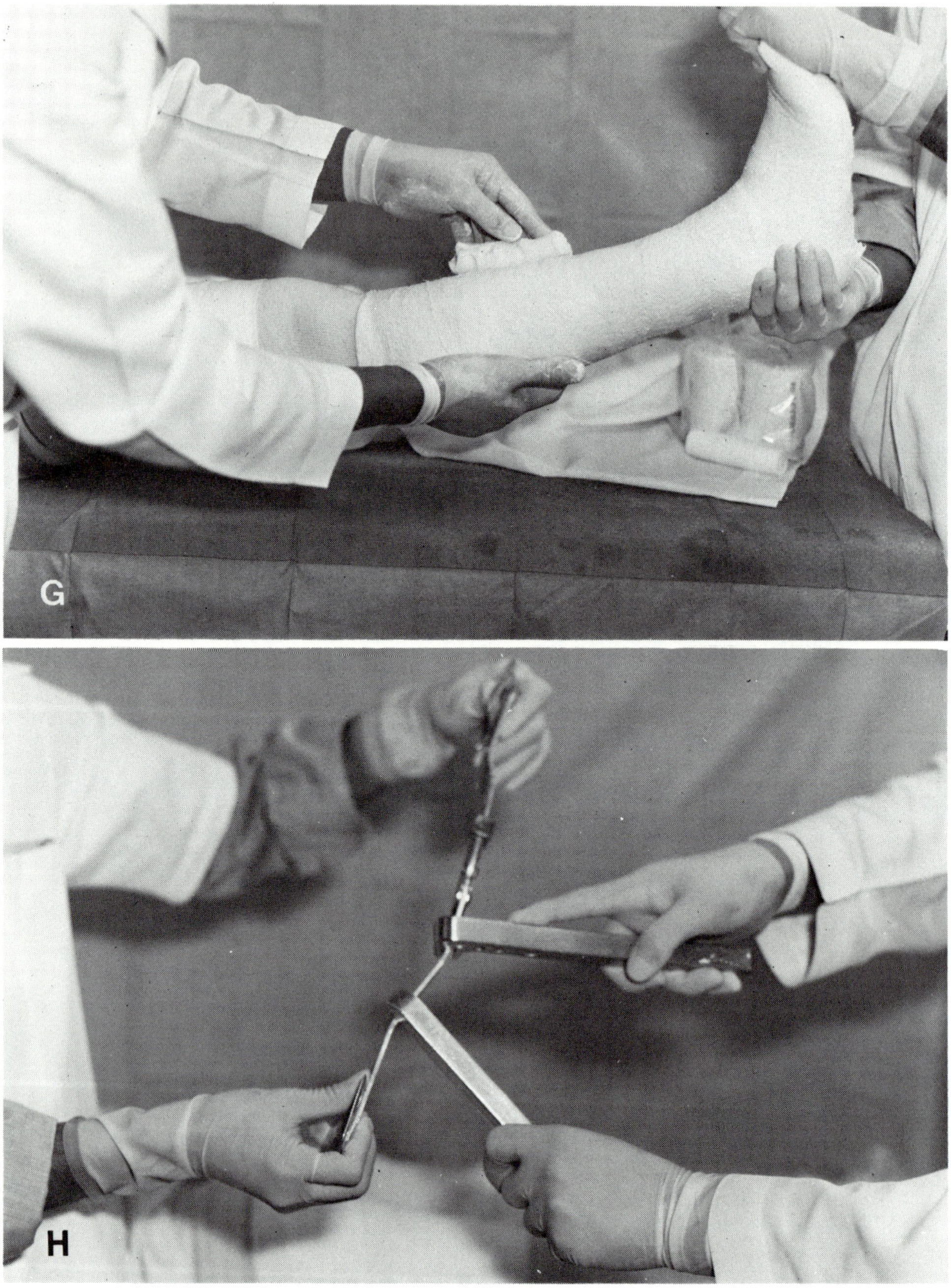

Fig. 4-10, continued. (G) Completion of the two segments of cast. One is a short-leg cast, including the foot, with the ankle in neutral position, and the other covers the quadrilateral plastic shell. *(H)* Bending the hinges to conform to the margins of the cast. *(Legend continued on opposite page.)*

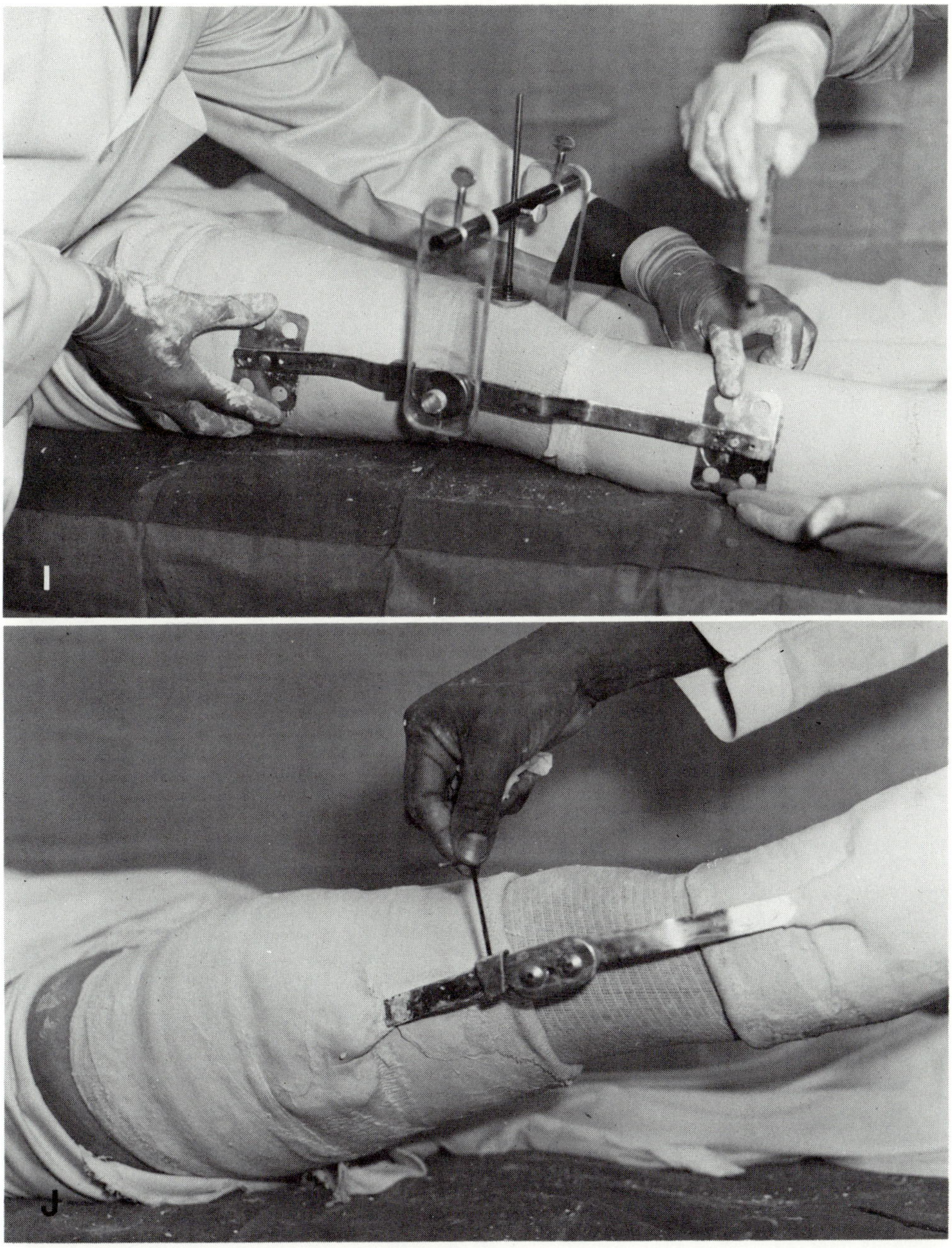

Fig. 4-10, continued. (I) Placing the hinges, using the template for proper alignment, being certain that the centers of rotation are equal and that they are in the same sagittal plane. *(J)* The hinge applied to the two segments of the cast. An Allen wrench locks the cast in extension, but the cast may be released and pulled proximally for bending. *(Legend continued on overleaf.)*

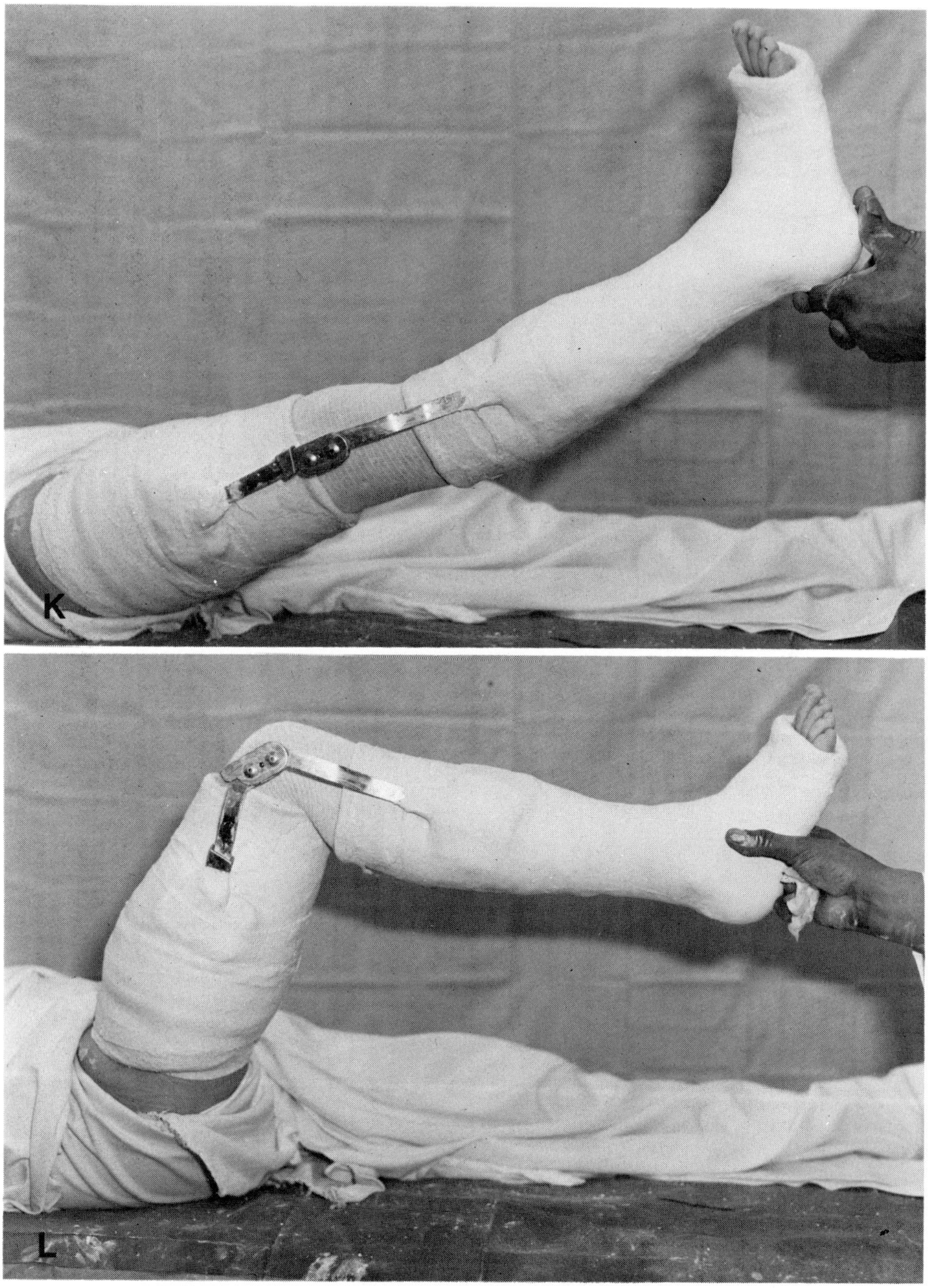

Fig. 4-10, continued. (K) The amount of extension that is possible with a cast brace. *(L)* The amount of flexion that is possible with a cast brace. Notice that the posterior portion is cut high enough to allow 90 degrees of flexion at the knee. *(Legend continued on opposite page.)*

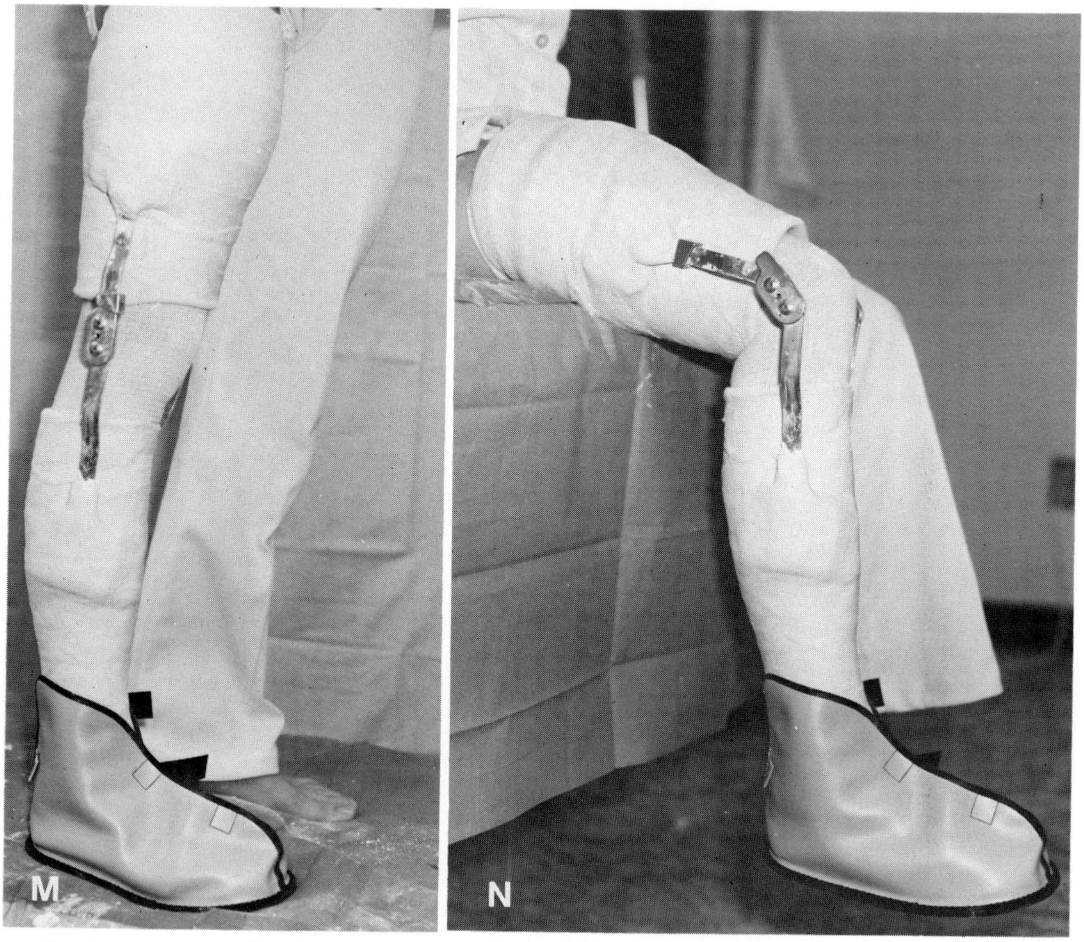

Fig. 4-10, continued. (M) The patient standing with a cast shoe and the brace in full extension. *(N)* The patient sitting with the knee bent to a comfortable angle.

Actual treatment of the fracture depends upon the specific case involved. The reader is referred to the voluminous literature concerning this subject. The cast brace, however, appears to be a very useful tool. The well-rounded practitioner or cast technician should be versed in its application.

CAST CARE

Once the cast has been properly applied, the patient should be instructed concerning care of the cast.

Prevention of Wetting

The first and foremost precaution should be against allowing the cast to become wet or damp. This is particularly important in cases of walking casts when dampness occurs from walking in wet grass or weeds or on wet streets or sidewalks. Many patients ask permission to take a bath with a cast on, using a plastic bag to protect the cast from water. It is best to advise against immersion of the cast in a bathtub filled with water, even with a plastic bag, since many times leakage does occur particularly around in the top of the bag, and the cast inadvertently becomes wet. Wetness will destroy the hardness of the cast and will make the plaster begin to fragment and break so that the cast will be destroyed. The cast can be cleansed with a damp cloth, provided the primary purpose is to remove surface soil from the cast. Most of the time, careful surface cleansing can be accomplished without difficulty. In areas where staining has occurred, touch-up of the cast with white shoe polish will make the cast more presentable.

Prevention of Odors

A problem with many casts is that an odor develops due to retention of perspiration and body oils in the cast. As the body secretions or wound drainage are absorbed into the cast padding and ultimately into the cast itself, it begins to impart a very foul odor. This may become so objectionable as to require a complete change of cast. Commercial deodorants are available to incorporate into the cast at the time of application, but these are not usually effective. In previous years, the addition of charcoal and chlorophyll compounds was advised for use in casts, particularly in those that covered areas in which wound drainage was anticipated. These additives have not proved greatly effective, and most are no longer in use.

Prevention of Skin Irritation

Care should be taken to avoid skin irritation under the cast. Particularly, this includes prevention of scratching with foreign objects under the cast. Many people will make an attempt to scratch the area of skin with a long metallic object which is slipped under the cast to quiet an aggravating itching sensation. This is to be strictly prohibited. Many times, an actual breaking of the skin will occur with subsequent cast sore formation. The same applies to the introduction of various other materials under the cast. The use of deodorant sprays and other aerosol-propelled medications under the cast is to be discouraged, since it will often result in an irritation or breaking out of the skin. It is permissible to apply small amounts of talcum powder or corn starch under the cast to provide some comfort to the skin and promote drying, particularly when excessive perspiration is a problem. Deodorant powders may be sprinkled under a cast, provided the patient has been specifically tested for sensitivity to the preparation.

Prevention of Softening

Softening of the cast, particularly at the heel, from resting the cast on the floor is almost invariably present and is of little consequence. The bearing of weight on the undersurface of the cast without protection is to be prevented since this softens the cast and destroys its effectiveness. The patient is encouraged to take care of the cast and to report to the physician any breaks or abnormal softenings, so that repairs can be done and the effectiveness of the cast can be maintained.

CAST REMOVAL

Probably few things have meant as much to the intern and the junior orthopaedic resident as has the development of the mechanical cast saw. Prior to 1945, casts were removed by a various group of instruments known as "cast cutters." These were devices which depended upon the manual crushing or breaking of a trough through the cast with long lever arms in order to create a defect in the side of the cast. Not only did this require a great amount of exertion on the part of the physician or technician removing the cast, but also it was a difficult, painful procedure for the patient forced to endure this primitive and time-consuming ordeal.

The invention of the cast saw, however, makes removal of casts a very easy and convenient procedure that can be accomplished in a relatively short period of time with comfort to the patient. As a general rule, the cast is removed by "bivalving." This simply means cutting the cast in a longitudinal manner in the midlateral space on either side (Fig. 4-11). This then allows the cast to be split, and the top, or front half, removed so that the extremity can be lifted out of the posterior shell. This can be done quite easily, but care should be taken when the front half is removed that the extremity is not unduly moved or manipulated by the stockinett or cast padding that is attached both to the cast and to the extremity. Once the soft elements of the padding have been cut through with a pair of scissors, the front half of the cast can be removed quite easily and the extremity can be left in the posterior shell for subsequent removal or transport to the x-ray department. The posterior shell can be removed periodically for physical therapy, hot soaks at home, or change of dressing over wounds. After removal of the cast, walking heels, walking irons, or metal hinges from cast braces can be salvaged and, if in good condition, used again.

CAST CHANGES

Indications

The indications for change of cast are, for the most part, medical and at the discretion of the attending physician. As a general rule, if the cast has become soft or otherwise structurally unsound to the extent that it cannot be repaired, a cast change is indicated. In children, growth of the extremity necessitates the periodical change of casts to allow for increased size.

Casts are occasionally changed because they have become loose. This may be due to atrophy of the underlying muscle, cast padding that has been used so that it no longer is as thick as it was, or the loss of edema fluid. Attempts at reducing the size of the cast without changing it are usually futile; it is much better to change the cast and apply a smaller, more snugly fitting one than to try to "take up" a cast that is too large. The new cast can be molded again to fit the contour of the extremity. If the fracture is so recent that solidarity has not been achieved great care must be taken at the time of cast change to prevent loss of reduction. In fact, it is better to make whatever arrangements are necessary to avoid a change of cast until a certain amount of "stickiness" of the fracture has occurred.

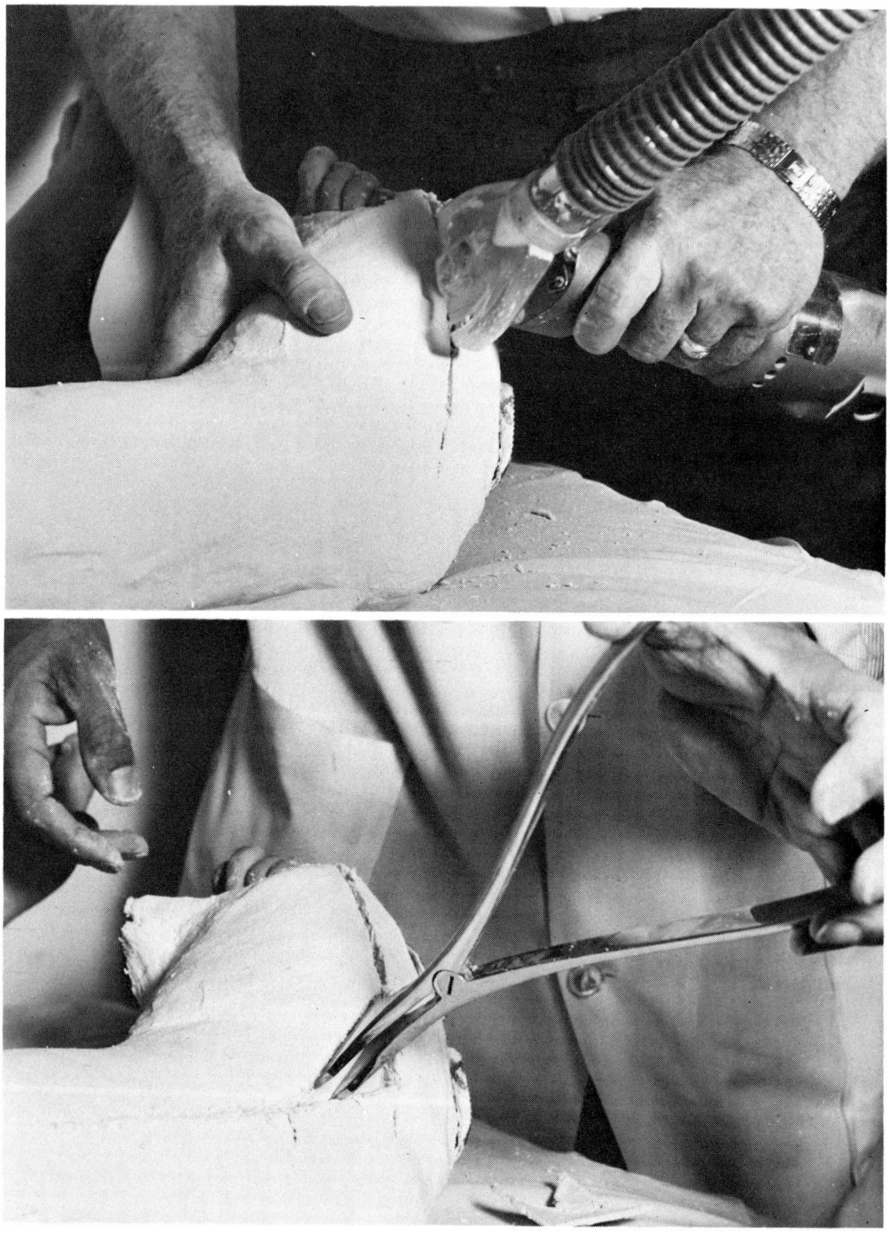

Fig. 4-11. (This page and opposite) Bivalving. The cast is split into two sections, one anterior and one posterior. In the case of a short-leg cast, a small triangular defect is created at the angle of the ankle, so that spreaders may be introduced. Holding the leg in position to the posterior part of the cast the anterior part is removed with spreaders, the padding and stockinett are cut, and the leg is removed from the posterior shell. The posterior shell can be retained for use as a temporary splint, if desired, by attaching it to the leg with a circumferentially placed elastic bandage.

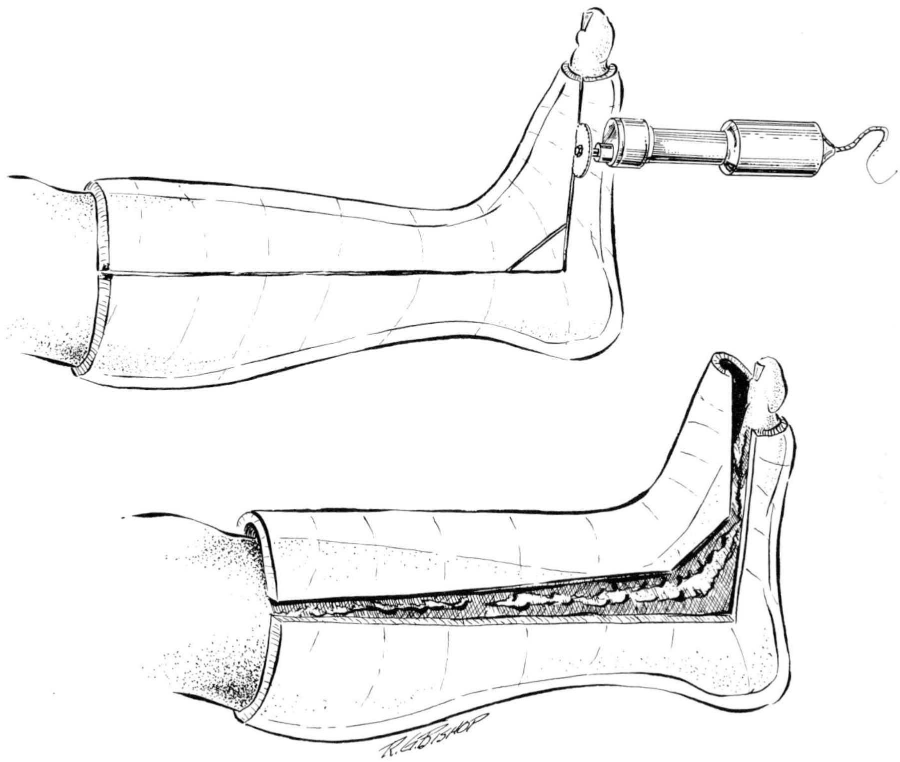

Fig. 4-11, continued.

Maintaining Position

When the cast is finally changed, under whatever circumstances, care must be taken to avoid undue stress on the fracture site; bowing might result even if the reduction is maintained in apposition. This is particularly true, for instance, in the case of lower extremity casts which are applied for immobilization of fractures of the tibia. If the leg is held horizontal to the table with the patient lying down, supporting it at the knee and the ankle, bowing of the tibia at the fracture site will sometimes occur due to the pull of gravity. When the cast is reapplied, this bowing is maintained in plaster. In instances when the fracture is not solid, it is much better to apply the cast with the patient sitting up so that the pull of gravity is along the longitudinal axis of the tibia with the leg hanging over the side of the table (Fig. 4-12), The cast can be applied without fear of bowing at the fracture site. Once the lower portion of the cast has been applied, the patient may lie down and the operator may apply the cast from the knee up. Even if the examiner is reasonably sure that the position of the fracture has been maintained after the change of cast, additional roentgenograms should be taken to document the fact that the fracture is still in position and to discover any changes in position that might have occurred without his realizing it. It should be a standard rule to recheck the position of all fractures in extremities which have had a cast change to be certain that no alteration of position has occurred.

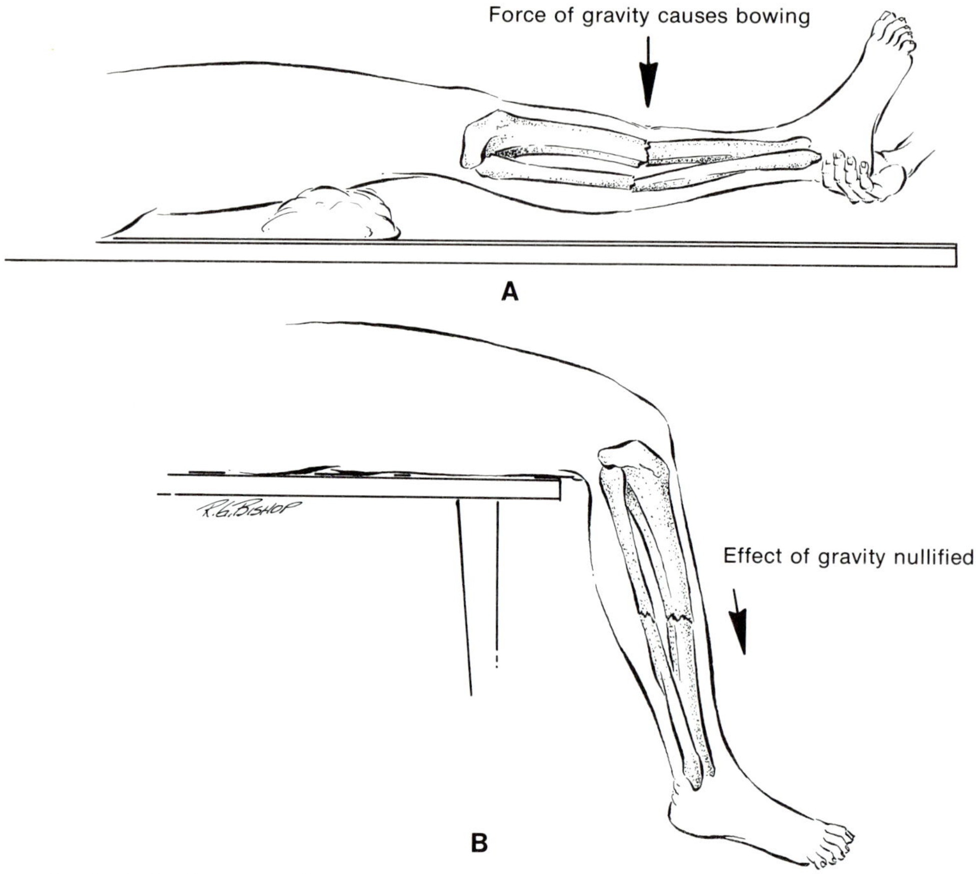

Fig. 4-12. At the time of cast change for fractures of the tibia, care must be taken to avoid bowing at the fracture site, even in a partially healed fracture. *(A)* If the leg is held suspended, the effect of gravity may cause a posterior bowing in an unstable fracture, due to the presence of fixed points at the knee and at the ankle, with the center being subjected to the pull of gravity. *(B)* If, however, the patient is placed on the side of the table with the leg hanging over the side, the effect of gravity is nullified, and the cast can be applied without fear of the posterior bowing.

Skin Care

Skin care should be done at the time of cast change or following removal of the cast. The skin under the cast is likely to accumulate a considerable amount of desquamated epithelium that has not been allowed to rub off under the normal processes of wear. It is interesting to note how much "dead skin" accumulates under a cast and to realize that desquamated epithelium was present over the remainder of the body, but was removed by constant friction against clothes, bed clothes, and the like. Under the cast this friction does not occur. The desquamated epithelium merely collects as an accumulation of a dirty, grey, sometimes foul-smelling skin (from the accumulation of rancid seborrheic material). The dead skin is still adherent to the underlying skin surface; attempts at scratching it off or rubbing it off by brisk movements will occasionally irritate the normal skin. Rashes and abraded areas offer some difficulty, particularly if a cast is to be reapplied. The patient should be cautioned against scratching an area of an extremity from which a cast has been removed. While this is particularly important in young children who do not know better, it is surprising how many adults subconsciously will begin to rub vigorously an extremity that has been removed from a cast, causing abraded areas on the very tender skin underlying this layer of desquamated epithelium. Rather than to remove this by friction, it is much better to wait until the extremity can be immersed in water. If the cast is to be reapplied, however, and if the stability of the fracture allows only minimal manipulation of the extremity, the skin may be cleansed by gentle sponging with a mild detergent or germicidal soap. Only that portion of the desquamated material that is readily loosened should be removed. All areas that are still adherent to the underlying skin should be left intact. Once the skin has been sponged off, the new cast can be reapplied with a degree of comfort. If the cast is removed permanently, the extremity can be immersed in a warm water bath with gentle sponging, again with a detergent or germicidal soap. Following drying (patting with a dry towel), the skin can be treated with some type of lanolin cream, lubrication cream, or lotion. This has a soothing effect upon the skin, it helps to restore some of the oiliness of the skin that has been lost to desiccation under the cast, and also it helps to remove desquamated epithelium. Some patients tend to have a much greater accumulation of epithelium than others. In some cases, it requires several treatments to remove all of the desquamated epithelium from the extremity.

Special mention should be made of the development of skin rashes under a cast. In patients who perspire abundantly, the skin sometimes remains somewhat macerated under the cast. A skin rash that resembles "prickly heat" will be seen. This sometimes becomes severe enough to necessitate removal of the cast. In other instances, the rash will develop secondary infection from resident skin bacteria that multiply in the moist environment; multiple pustules will form, particularly in hair follicles. These pustules may develop into large local reactions and may necessitate either removal of the cast or extensive windowing in order to expose them to the air. Severe rashes that occur under the cast are best treated by exposure to the air and by removal of the covering that has produced the excessive accumulation of perspiration and skin debris. At times this is very difficult to do. The instability of the fracture may necessitate institution of balanced traction for a period of time until the skin can be cleared up and the cast reapplied. Skin rashes may result from sensitivity to the cast material or to medications included under the cast. Severe eczematoid reactions may occur, which likewise necessitate removal of the entire cast, or at least windowing with removal of a portion of the cast overlying the affected area. The treatment of rashes tests the ingenuity of the practitioner. One is torn between the need to maintain support of the fresh fracture and the need to uncover the area of skin reaction in order for it to heal. If the skin rash continues to be severe, consultation with a dermatologist is indicated.

WINDOWS

The advent of the oscillating-blade cast saw, which allowed a longitudinal thin saw cut through the plaster cast, immediately opened the possibilities for creating windows in casts. Any area can be removed by marking off a square or rectangular area and cutting along the lines. This segment can then be removed so that the underlying skin can be exposed. The windows provide several important advantages. First, they enable the practitioner to examine an area under the cast, particularly a surgical wound. The surgical wound that has been covered by a cast should be inspected occasionally to be certain that healing is occurring without difficulty and that no evidence exists of wound infection. It is necessary, also, to expose surgical wounds to remove sutures once healing has been accomplished. It has become popular in recent years to close surgical wounds that will be covered by a cast with skin tapes rather than with sutures. This obviates suture removal at a later date. However, it is wise to create a small window over the operative area for inspection of the wound 2 or 3 weeks postoperatively, to be certain that all is well with the wound. If it is found that the wound is satisfactory, the window can be replaced easily and the cast repaired over the area.

Windows also are important for removal of pins that have been left protruding from the extremity when they have been utilized for fixation devices. Occasionally an unstable fracture of the tibia can be held with a single diagonally placed pin drilled across the fracture site to maintain position until some healing of the fracture can be accomplished. The pin is left extending through the skin and is removed as soon as enough healing has occurred so that apposition will be maintained. It is important that these pins be inspected periodically to be certain that migration is not occurring. It is important also that the pins not be covered with a circumferential cast. The cast may put continual pressure on the end of the pin and may drive it further into the extremity. When pins are left protruding, a small window can be made over the end of the pin. The patient can be asked to inspect the pin daily to be certain that migration does not occur.

In hands, it is many times necessary to have Kirschner wires drilled into the bone to stabilize joints, and small fragments of bone, or to otherwise immobilize portions of the hand. The hand is occasionally also placed in a plaster cast to help make the stability more secure. In these instances, the pins must be inspected periodically to be certain that they are not driven further into the hand. They are quite small and sharp and easily may be driven further into the hand with continuous or repeated pressure on the protruding end of the pin. The window that is cut over the pin may be small and should be filled with a small sponge rubber or polyfoam pad into which the pin can protrude. The window can then be replaced and taped into position.

Another indication for windowing a cast is the presence of symptoms suggesting a pressure area on the skin. This has been covered in some detail in the section dealing with cast application, but it is important to point out that the cutting of a window in the cast over a pressure area will often relieve the pressure area. If, however, the window is left open, the skin in the area uncovered by the window will have a tendency to swell through the window and to form pressure areas around the margins of the window (Fig. 4-13). This can be prevented by cutting a small plastic foam pad the exact size of the window, cutting the cotton padding away from the area, and inserting the foam plastic pad to cover the area of skin that has been exposed. The plaster shell comprising the window can then be replaced to hold the foam pad in place. The plastic foam will not only prevent localized swelling from occurring in the area of

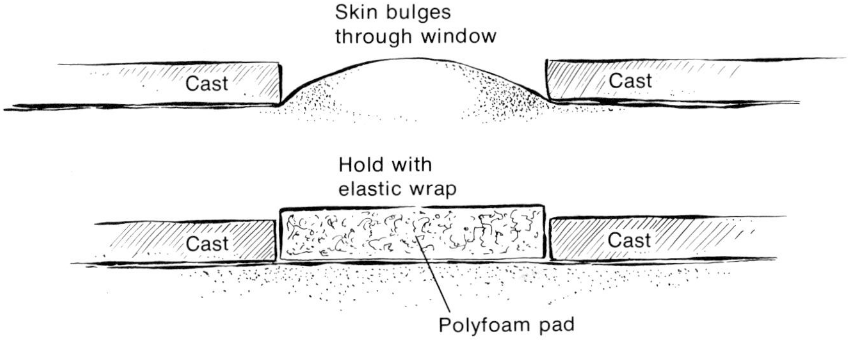

Fig. 4-13. When a window is cut in a cast, either over a swollen area or a wound, there is a tendency for the skin to bulge through the window *(A)*. Swelling generally is controlled by the cast itself, but in the area of a window the swelling goes uncontrolled, and there results blistering or damage to the skin along the margins of the cast. *(B)* This can be eliminated by the application of a polyfoam pad in the window. The pad should be cut to the precise size of the window, so that it can be placed in the window and held with an elastic wrap. This creates a counterpressure that prevents swelling and the extrusion of soft tissue through the open window. The pad can be removed periodically for inspection of the area exposed, and reapplied as necessary.

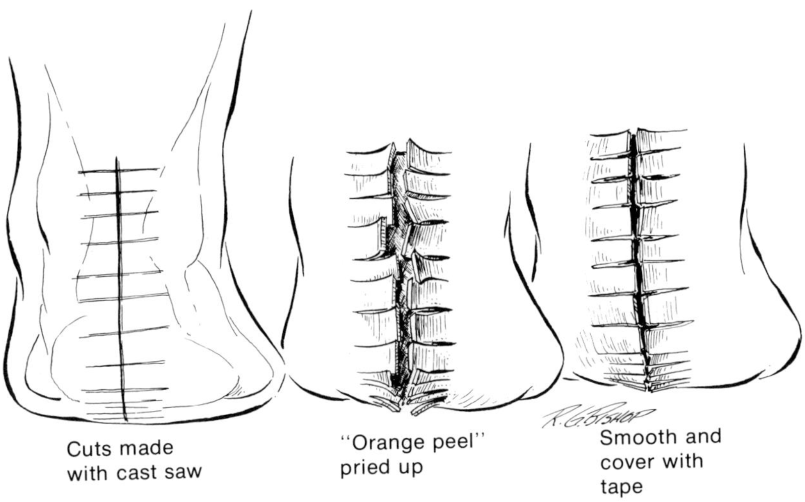

Fig. 4-14. Orange peeling can be used to eliminate pressure areas, particularly over the heel or over other bony prominences. A longitudinal cut is made with the cast saw directly over the pressure area. Crosscuts are made at right angles to the longitudinal cut, at approximately ½-cm. intervals. This results in numerous small segments of cast that are still hinged at the margin but are free in the center. These can be bent out to expose the underlying tissue. The tissue can then be examined, the padding can be removed if necessary, and the cast can be pushed back into place, but there is a much softer contour due to the bending and softening of the cast accomplished by the orange peeling maneuver. The area of orange peeling is then covered with adhesive tape in order to hold it in position.

exposed tissue, but also will relieve the pressure phenomenon by substituting the softness of plastic foam for the hardness of the cast wall.

In the case of pressure areas over the heel, the same technique can be used. It is better, however, to substitute a technique called "orange peeling" to relieve the pressure and to prevent pressure from occurring around the margins of the window. "Orange peeling" is a technique whereby a longitudinal cut is made with the saw blade directly over the heel; at right angles to the cut and transversely across it, multiple saw cuts are made approximately 4 mm. apart extending a centimeter or so across on either side of the cut. This portion of the cast is pried up and it becomes completely soft and yielding. This also prevents swelling through the window and softens the pressure area (Fig. 4-14).

Windows are sometimes cut in casts to expose areas of skin reaction or skin rash. Multiple windows may be cut in large casts to allow for circulation of air and its cooling effect.

Whatever the indication for removing a window, care must be taken that the structural integrity of the cast is not altered.

CORRECTIVE CASTS

The basic function of the casting technique is the maintanence of position of an extremity when definitive treatment of the fracture has been accomplished. The cast represents a mechanism for immobilizing and holding the reduced fracture rather than correcting the fracture. It is well known that attempts to use casts for the correction of position in fracture treatment have resulted in pressure sore formation and in vascular disturbances because of the inability of the average cast to do the dynamic correction itself. It would follow that the vast majority of casts are not considered corrective casts *per se*. The number of instances in which the cast is used as a correcting device is relatively limited.

Club Foot Casts

One of those instances in which casting can be considered to be corrective casting is in the treatment of club foot and similar conditions of childhood and infancy. In these cases, however, the cast itself does not actually constitute the correcting mechanism, but merely is the agent by which the correction is maintained. The cast technique described by Kite in the treatment of club foot deformities has the cast applied in sections. The cast is used as a mechanism for holding the forefoot, and ultimately the hindfoot, while the correction is established manually and the remainder of the cast is applied. The cast itself does not constitute the dynamic correcting force, but merely serves to hold the foot once the correction has been established. It would appear to be a matter of semantics as to whether or not these constitute corrective casts. By the general definition of the term, the club foot cast is considered a true "corrective cast."

Wedged Casts

Another corrective cast is the wedged cast. Wedging is used when closed reduction of a fracture has resulted in restoration of apposition, but where some angular deformity still exists at the fracture site. A cast of a circular nature is applied to the extremity and allowed to harden. A wedged mechanism is created at the fracture site to correct the angulation or bowing. The

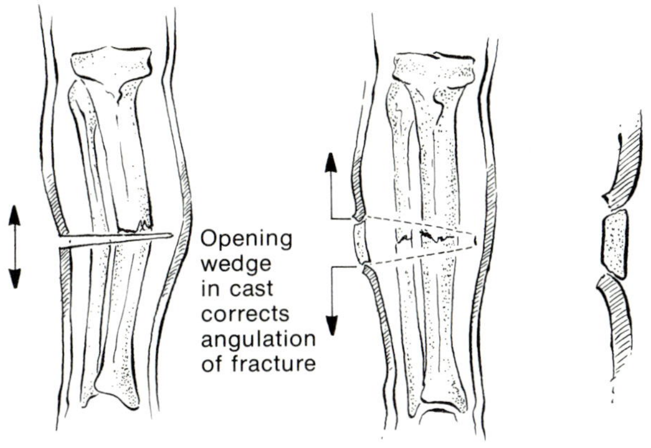

Fig. 4-15. Wedging of a cast is necessary to correct angulation at the fracture site in long bones. The saw cut is made at the angle of the fracture, extending from the concave side of the cast, and leaving a bridge of at least 2 cm. on the convex side. The cut should be made completely around the cast, except for the small hinge. The wedge is opened to correct the angulation of the fracture. The amount of angulation to be corrected is the determining factor in deciding how much to spread the defect. The margins of the cast at the defect are bent outward to prevent impingement on the skin. They are held apart by a roll of sheet wadding that has been prepared to hold the wedge satisfactorily, while an additional roll of plaster is placed circumferentially around the cast and wadding. Of course, roentgenograms should be taken immediately following this procedure, and additional correction should be done, if necessary. The wedge can be released slightly if overcorrection has occurred. The wedge should be held firmly in the corrected position until the circumferential plaster has completely set and has incorporated into the original plaster.

technique consists of making a transverse cut with the oscillating saw, extending around most of the circumference of the cast, but leaving a small hinge present on the *convex* side of the angulation. The saw cut extends entirely through the full thickness of the cast and leaves only a small segment of uncut cast on the convex side (Fig. 4-15). It is then possible to bend the cast at this level and open up the space at the point of the saw cut, utilizing the intact portion of cast as a hinge. This creates a wedge-shaped space, with its base formed on the convex side of the angulation. The correction is obtained by forcing the distal fragment forward into a corrected position by opening the wedge in the cast. Relatively large degrees of angulation can be corrected, as long as the apposition is good and no appreciable offset exists at the fracture site. Once the correction has been obtained and confirmation obtained by roentgenogram or image intensifier, the wedge is held open while additional plaster is applied to hold it in this corrected position.

Some operators prefer to insert a small block of wood or piece of plaster to hold the wedge open in the corrected position. This, however, has the danger of allowing the block or wedge to migrate into a position next to the skin, which might result in a pressure sore; therefore, it is better merely to hold the extremity in the corrected position while the margins of the wedge are bent slightly with the alligator forceps so that no chance of impingement of the cast margin on the skin can occur. The intervening space, or defect, is then filled in with a small piece of cast padding, and a plaster roll is used to hold the cast in this corrected position. The circumferentially placed roll of plaster extending above and below the wedge holds the cast in the corrected position, so that forcing the wedge open with a block of wood is not necessary. Care must be taken in this technique that no pressure areas exist under the cast, either at the margins of the wedge on the convex side or at the point of the hinge on the concave side of the fracture.

A modification of this technique involves removing a precalculated-size wedge of cast on the convex side of the fracture. This allows a closing of the wedge after removing the portion of plaster; again, a small strip of plaster is left on the concave side of the fracture to act as a hinge. This technique allows for a more stable situation, since the wedge is closed rather than open at the end of the correction. However, it is more likely to result in impingement of the cast on the underlying extremity; special care must be taken to avoid impingement if the closed wedge technique is used. In either event, the correction can be made and maintained by holding the extremity in the corrected position. Either of these techniques is recommended in instances in which angulation with good apposition occurs following closed reduction of a fracture. The wedged cast cannot be construed as being a dynamic correction by the cast, but most people continue to consider the wedged cast a corrective cast in the true sense of the word.

Dynamic Casts

There are some instances in which a dynamic correction is obtained by the use of special casting. An example of this is the hinge cast where a metallic hinge is incorporated into the cast with its mechanism falling at the apex of the spinal curve. The portion of cast incorporating the trunk, above and below, transforms these two areas into single lever arms. As the cast is pulled into position to the hinge, the angulation of the spine is corrected. Sometimes elastic-band traction is applied so that the cast has a dynamic corrective action and can be considered a true corrective cast.

Similar casts are used in correction of deformities of the hand and wrist. The cast is applied in a segmental manner with a hinge in the center, between the two segments. Outriggers then may be fashioned so that continuous gentle pull by elastic bands occurs to overcome the fibrous tissue contracture of the joint. Casts of this nature have mostly been supplanted by splints, which not only have the same dynamic action for correction with elastic band traction, but also have the additional feature that they can be removed for hydrotherapy, manual stretching, and other physical therapy.

5 Casts Other Than Plaster-of-Paris

Though the original concept of rigid padded fixation was developed following the advent of plaster-of-paris bandages, there have been reports of other materials used for fixation of extremities. To date, none of these has supplanted the original concept of casts made from plaster of paris. With continued development, however, it may be that the future will find other materials for rigid fixation which have advantages over plaster of paris without some of the disadvantages. At present, there are two materials used for casts other than plaster of paris. These include fiberglass materials and the opaque, white, thermolabile cast materials.

FIBERGLASS CASTS

Fiberglass casts that were introduced some 20 or 30 years ago required the addition of an acetone solvent to allow for their application and molding to the extremity. While these casts were lightweight, allowed the free flow of air through them and were impervious to water, the disadvantage was the frequent development of allergic reactions to the solvent. After the application of one of these casts, the patient's skin often developed a severe eczemoid rash which made removal of the cast necessary. These early attempts at the use of fiberglass casts have led to development of newer casts which have retained the advantagees of the old fiberglass cast and have eliminated the basic disadvantage.

The recently developed light-cured casts have been widely accepted. The material is applied to the extremity in a manner similar to that of application of plaster of paris. Following complete application of the bandage, the extremity is brought under an ultraviolet light, which cures the material and causes it to solidify into a hard, water-impervious cast. These casts have many of the advantages that were seen with the early fiberglass casts, in that they are lightweight, very tough and wear-resistant, and relatively radiolucent. They allow for more flow of air through the cast material since they are not completely homogeneous, as is plaster of paris. They have the added advantage that they are fast-drying; they are immediately hard enough to allow for early weightbearing. One of the advantages that is expounded by the developer and manufacturer is that the cast material is impervious to water. The cast and the extremity may be immersed in water without ill-effects to the cast itself. This is in contradistinction to plaster of paris, which becomes weakened and breaks readily when softened by wetting. The water-resistant feature is said to allow immersion of the cast when taking a bath or in the whirlpool when treating open wounds exposed by cast windows.

A word of caution, however, concerns wetting procedures. While it is true that the cast itself is impervious to water and is not effected by immersion, it should be remembered that the skin is wet within the cast; lack of air to dry the skin could permit maceration of the skin under the cast.

One must be careful to select padding material that will not retain water. Following immersion in water, one also must be careful to dry thoroughly under the cast with a hair dryer or similar apparatus once the cast has been dried. Failure to secure adequate drying of the skin after the extremity is removed from the water will result in serious skin changes that may even require removal of the cast.

Another disadvantage is difficulty in using the cast for fresh fractures which require manual holding to maintain position while the cast is drying. This is extremely difficult, if not impossible, with this type of cast. Therefore, the cast is recommended more for the subsequent cast changes following partial healing of the fracture than it is for the original casting following reduction of the fracture. Another disadvantage is the necessity of curing the cast under the special light supplied with the cast material. It is difficult to cure extremely large casts under the light because of the space limitations. It can be seen that if this cast is used exclusively in a busy orthopaedic practice, it may cause a bottleneck, since each of the casts has to cure for a specified time. Finally, the hardness of the cast makes it difficult to remove with the cast cutter; a special blade is necessary to cut through this extremely hard material. The blade must be changed often in order to maintain its cutting ability.

If one takes all of these factors into account, however, one can see that there still are advantages in using the fiberglass cast in selected cases. While most busy orthopaedists are not likely to use it as a routine casting material, there are probably instances in which its advantages far outweigh its disadvantages.

THERMOLABILE PLASTIC CASTS

A second type of cast material utilizes a thermolabile plastic material which has been manufactured as a mesh and dispensed in convenient-sized rolls. The rolls are dipped in hot water. They become quite malleable and can be applied to the extremity with considerable ease. The heating of the plastic material makes it adhere to itself quite readily; it becomes well-molded as it coalesces with other portions of the cast. Once cooling has occurred, which is relatively rapid, the cast becomes quite hard. It exhibits many of the characteristics described above for fiberglass casts. The material is strong, it is water-resistant, radiopaque, and light-weight. It has the same disadvantages as fiberglass. One advantage that this material has over the fiberglass is that heating of the cast will allow for some change in position, since it restores the malleability of the material. Position or contour can be changed slightly and the new position held as the material cools once again.

Both fiberglass and thermolabile plastic are bought at a relatively high cost at present. Of course, the cost may decrease as the popularity increases and volume sales allow for price reduction. The ill-effects to skin after immersion of these casts in water constitute their greatest disadvantage. If one is careful to prevent skin breakdown, however, fiberglass and thermolabile casts can be useful.

6 Splints

The word "splint" signifies the use of an apparatus that is not cylindrical and that lies along one or more surfaces of an extremity. It is a coaptive apparatus that is bound snugly to the extremity either by external binding material, such as an elastic bandage, or by some innate feature of the design of the splint itself. The splint is not free-standing, as is a cast, and it will not maintain its position next to the extremity without some mechanism to hold it on. This feature renders the splint much more adaptable; it can be molded to various contours, can be molded into various positions, and can be held to the extremity by a variety of wraps, straps, and outriggers extending from the splint itself. The splint is made of some rigid or semi-rigid substance. It can be made of plaster of paris so that after drying it becomes completely hard and unyielding, and the extremity must remain in exact position against it. It can be made of metal, which is as rigid, but is not as malleable as plaster. It also is not as form fitting as plaster. Plaster is molded to the contours of the extremity while still wet and allowed to set in the exact form desired. Metal splints are manufactured along certain general lines and cannot provide the fit that other splint materials provide. As a result, their use is strictly limited. Finally, the advent of the newer plastic materials has created a large variety of materials which are readily adaptable to the manufacture of splints.

While some of the plastic materials are as hard as plaster or metal, others are more resilient and allow for a certain amount of motion, even when applied snugly to the extremity. Most of the malleable plastics have some mechanism for providing malleability, but revert to the rigid or semi-rigid state when in use. The best known mechanism for making the splint malleable is heat. These materials become quite soft and malleable when heated; they can be applied to the extremity and molded to follow the contour very closely. Once the material has cooled, however, it becomes rigid and holds the shape. The plastic materials provide the advantages of the plaster fixation without the disadvantages inherent in plaster-of-paris appliances. They afford the same rigidity as plaster of paris and the same malleability, but they also are impervious to water. They can be washed, and they resist the effect of secretions from open wounds. Drainage from wounds can be washed off and the padding can be removed, while plaster-of-paris splints absorb drainage and may become quite objectionable. The newer plastic materials may become the most popular splint materials. Though they require some experience and practice to become expert in their use, to the experienced practitioner they probably provide the cleanest and most effective method of splinting.

PURPOSE

Basically, splints are applied either to provide immobilization for the extremity or to provide correction. Immobilization is doubtlessly its most popular application. The splint can immobilize an extremity for anything from photography of the extremity to improvement of the extremity's functional capability. For use as a corrective device, the splint has been so fashioned and so equipped with additional apparatus that it provides a certain correction for either deformities of the extremity or for functional motor loss. In these cases, the splint is usually a dynamic corrector, but it also can be a static corrector. The splint sometimes is made for nighttime wear to preserve correction that has been obtained by other means. In these instances, the splint is neither considered truly an immobilizer nor is it considered truly a corrective device; its function lies somewhere in between.

Splints for Immobilization

The splint that is used for immobilization is basically designed to fit the extremity well and to maintain the desired position once it has been applied. Most splints used for immobilization are arranged in such a manner that they can be removed periodically for physical therapy, for dressing change, or for other procedures.

The immobilization is not as perfect as it is in the circular cast or plaster bandage, since splints encompass only one joint. Immobilization of the entire extremity by a splint alone usually is not possible. An exception is the airplane splint which is used to immobilize the shoulder in abduction. Here the remainder of the extremity is immobilized because it must be held in a certain relationship with the body. For the most part, splints are used for the portions of the extremity distal to the elbow and knee joint, and are used when somewhat less than complete immobilization is indicated. Some splints actually are used to immobilize the elbow or knee joint, but seldom is an effective splint made which will immobilize the hip.

Readymade Splints. Almost all surgical equipment companies supply "readymade" splints for use on the upper or lower extremities. These are made either of metal, metal with plastic coating, or of plastic alone. They conform rather roughly to the shape of the extremity and come in various sizes so that some semblance of fit can be made. These readymade splints, however, cannot hope to afford a very good fit of the extremity since they are for general use. The old adage that "a splint is made to fit *everybody* so that it does not fit *anybody* very well" is a true one. Most readymade splints are roughly half circular in form, are of varied lengths, and roughly adhere to the contour of the extremity.

In the case of the upper extremity, there are long arm splints that extend from the axilla down to the hand, holding the elbow in varying degrees of flexion. There are short arm splints which extend from the elbow to the metacarpal-phalangeal junction and are used primarily for immobilization of the wrist or the distal portion of the forearm (Fig. 6-1).

Splints are made to fit the entire lower extremity, extending from the groin down to the tip of the foot, holding the knee in varying degrees of flexion and holding the ankle at a right angle. Again, these splints do not fit well and are

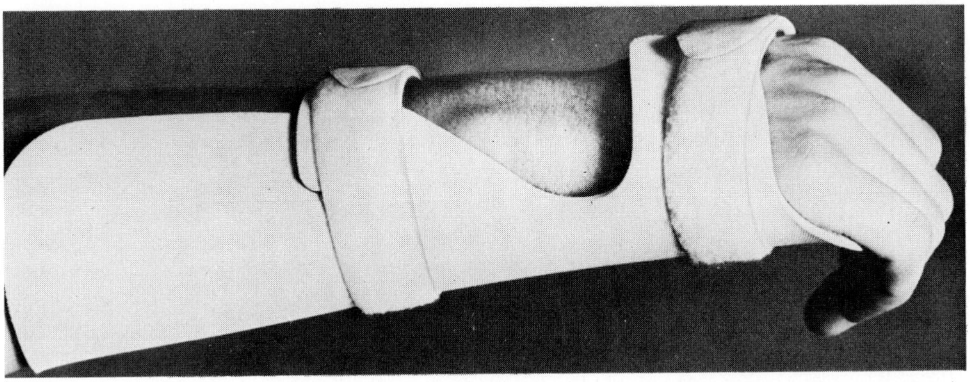

Fig. 6-1. A readymade wrist splint. (Courtesy of Thermo-Mold Medical Products, Inc.)

made for temporary immobilization. They are applied over a voluminous fluff or cotton dressing where the fit of the splint is of little importance. These splints are for temporary use and are replaced with a specially made splint which is made to fit the extremity very well.

Specially Made Splints. Specially made splints are made for perfect fitting to the extremity and are fashioned in such a way that they are quite malleable when applied. By the process of drying and cooling, they become rigid and fixed and adhere to the contour and position in which they are applied.

Splints are more useful when applied to the extremities distal to the elbow and knee and are particularly useful in the upper extremity for immobilization of the wrist and hand. When a single posterior splint extends from the gluteal crease to incorporate the entire lower extremity and foot, or when it extends from the axilla to incorporate the entire upper extremity including the elbow, wrist, and hand, some other type of splinting device should be substituted. The majority of splinting materials are not strong enough to withstand the pressure applied at the knee and at the elbow. There are special features for immobilization of the knee and elbow *per se* which have been featured by the Thermo-Mold Medical Products Company and will be described below. Other than this, however, splints for the lower extremity are basically short-leg splints for holding the tibia and ankle in neutral position. Adaptations for the upper extremity usually are in the form of short-arm splints designed to hold the wrist and forearm in a specified position.

Splints Can be Made of Plaster. Most companies that market plaster-of-paris bandages also market splints made of strips of crinoline and plaster in varying lengths and widths. They are packed in boxes of that configuration.

Plaster splints used in thicknesses of eight to 10 layers are encased in two layers of cast padding to prevent the plaster from coming in contact with the skin or the overlying bandage. The splint is trimmed on its margins to fit the contour of the extremity and molded while still wet around the extremity; it is held in place with a circular elastic bandage. As soon as the plaster has set, the splint can be removed and allowed to dry completely before it is reapplied (Fig. 6-2). When it is necessary for splints to encompass the entire length of the arm

(Text continued on page 114.)

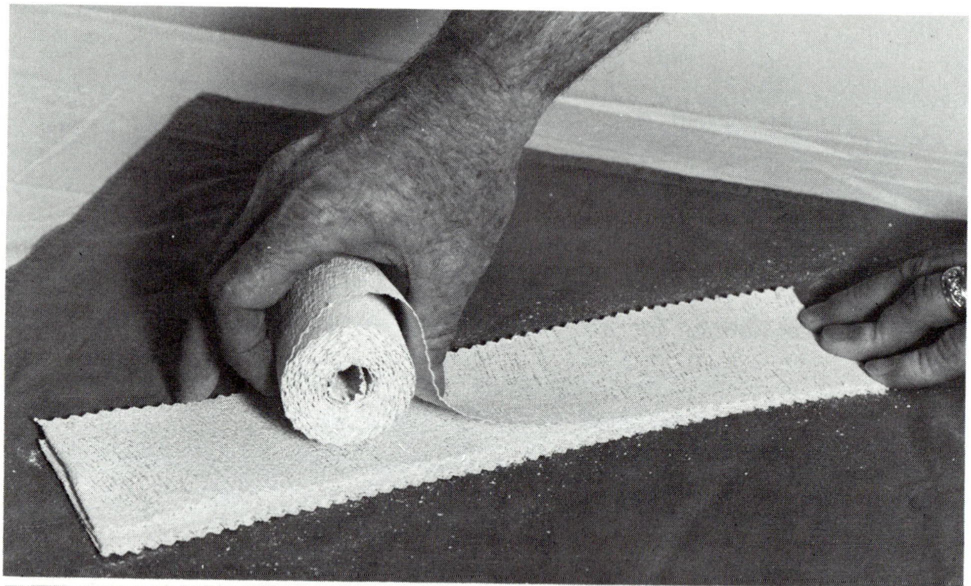

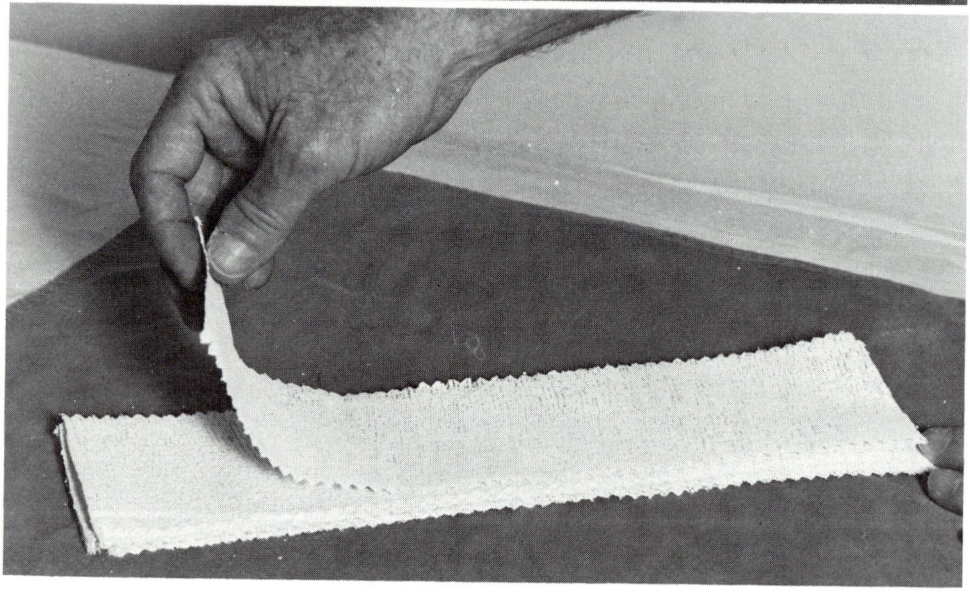

Fig. 6-2. (This page and opposite) Volar splint construction. Eight to ten thicknesses of plaster bandage are measured and assembled, dipped in water, squeezed as dry as possible, and then spread out and smoothed on cast padding. The padding is applied to both sides, and the splint is trimmed, leaving space for the thumb to move. The splint is then applied to the extremity, holding the hand and wrist in the corrected position. The splint is bound with an elastic bandage, which is kept in place until the splint has firmly set. The elastic bandage is then removed and reapplied at the proper amount of tension.

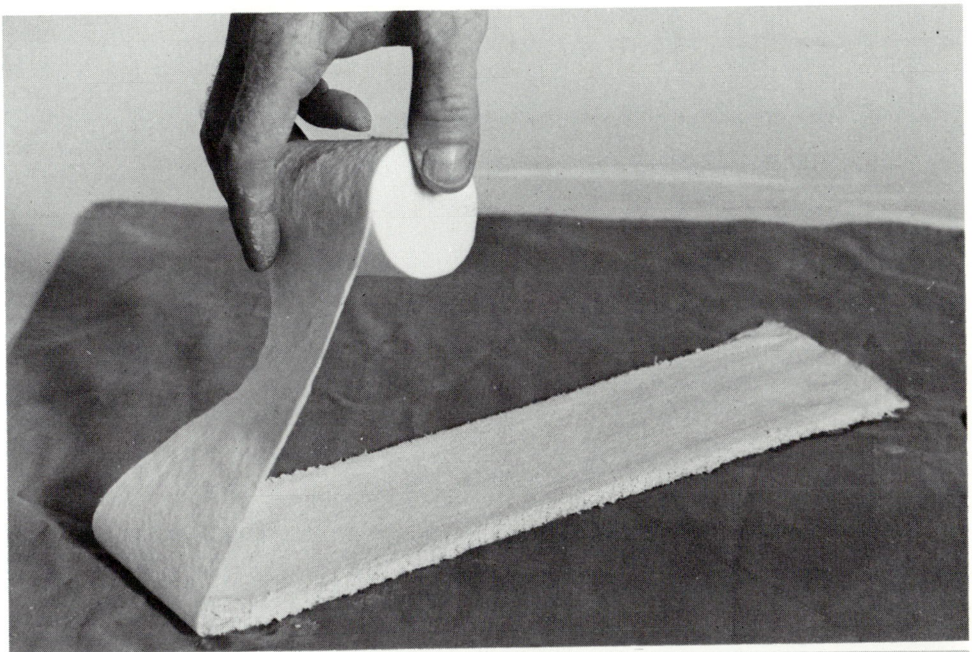

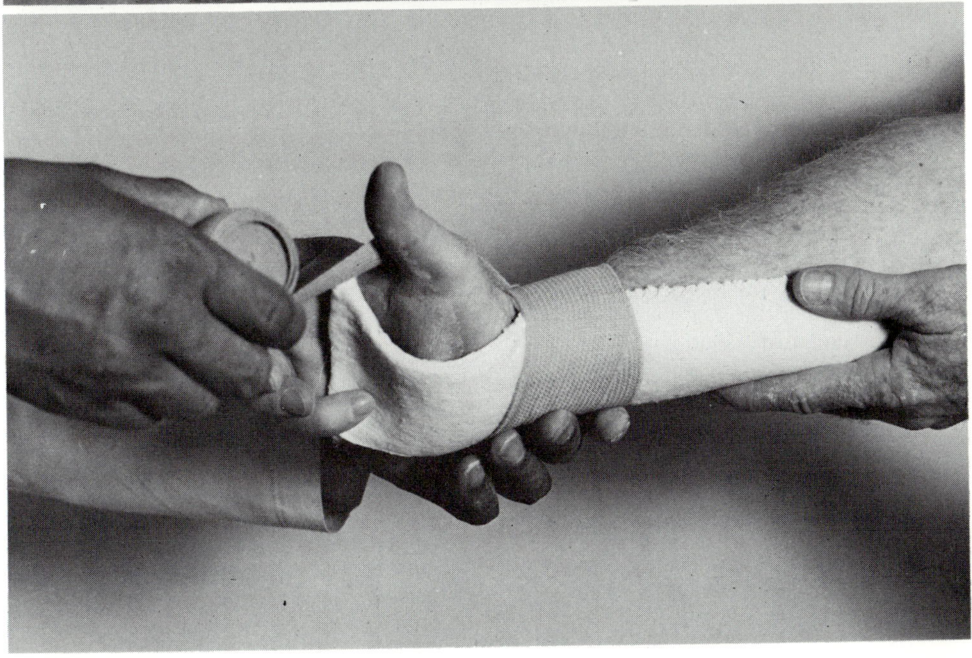

Fig. 6-2, continued.

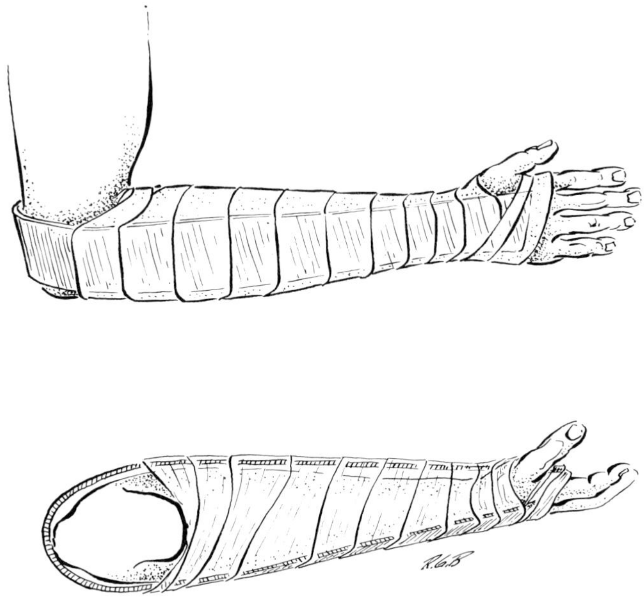

Fig. 6-3. The construction of a sugar-tong splint. The length of plaster required for the splint should be enough to reach from the proximal joints of the finger dorsally, across the dorsum of the wrist, around the elbow held at 90 degrees of flexion, and then up the volar side to extend to the distal flexion crease of the palm. A small slot is removed over the thenar eminence so that the thumb can be brought into better opposition. The cast is made of eight to ten thicknesses of plaster which are wet, squeezed as dry as possible, and spread out and smoothed on a hard surface. The splint is then covered on either side with cast padding and applied in the position described. It is held in place with elastic bandages, using a 3-inch elastic bandage for the elbow and forearm portion, and a 2-inch elastic bandage for the distal forearm, wrist, and hand. The wrist is held in the desired position while the plaster sets, and the elbow is maintained at as close to 90 degrees as possible. The sugar-tong splint prevents pronation and supination, gives firm immobilization to the wrist, and, at the same time, allows from 90 degrees flexion to 120 degrees extension at the elbow.

they may be reinforced at the elbow with additional splints that create a support across the bend and give additional strength. Otherwise, when applied entirely posteriorly, the splints are not strong enough to prevent motion at the elbow or at the knee.

A variation of the splint is used commonly for forearm and wrist fractures and is called the sugar-tong splint. The manufacture of this splint is demonstrated in Figure 6-3. The basic splint has been fashioned much as has been described for a volar splint except that the length is measured from the metacarpal heads, dorsally, and the strip passes over the dorsum of the wrist, forearm, and around the elbow, and passes on the volar side, extending past the wrist up to the distal flexion crease of the hand. The sugar-tong splint is made of eight or 10 thicknesses of plaster which are first wet and then squeezed relatively dry. The splint is smoothed out on a flat surface and is covered on either side with a layer of cast padding material. The area of the thenar eminence is cut out slightly with a pair of scissors or a scalpel blade, and the palmar surface is beveled slightly to fit the contour of the distal flexion crease of the palm. The splint is then applied with the elbow in approximately 90 degrees of flexion and the forearm in neutral supination-pronation. While in this position, the splint is extended from the metacarpal heads dorsally around the entire forearm to emerge on the palm at the distal flexion crease. A 3-inch elastic bandage is used to wrap the proximal portion of the splint, including the elbow and extending down onto the distal portion of the forearm. A 2-inch elastic bandage is used to extend from the distal portion of the forearm, past the wrist, onto the hand. The forearm is generally left in neutral supination–pronation, though occasionally some advantage can result from placing the forearm in either supination or pronation as the plaster splint dries. The position is dictated entirely by the condition being treated. When a Colles' fracture is being treated, it is necessary also to apply a slight amount of flexion at the wrist while the plaster is drying. This allows for a much more stable position of the radius in a Colles' fracture of the wrist. However, it is not the purpose of this text to dictate the position but merely to describe basic principles for the application of the splint and to relate its uses, advantages, and disadvantages. These specially made splints of plaster of paris, once dry, can be removed and reapplied as directed by the physician's orders.

Plastic Splints. In recent years, various casting materials have been developed which lend themselves very readily to the formation of splints. They have become quite popular. A material marketed by Johnson and Johnson Company as Orthoplast was the first to be developed and still enjoys wide popularity (Fig. 6-4). The material is dispensed in sheets. When cool, it forms a very hard, tough, plastic material which is very difficult to cut while in the rigid state. When the material is warmed in hot water, however, it becomes very soft and pliable and can be readily cut with bandage scissors and molded to fit the contours of the extremity during the cooling stage. While the material is still warm and malleable, the molding process can be accompanied by wrapping with a circumferential elastic bandage which holds the splint very snugly to the extremity while the plastic cools and hardens. Once cooling has occurred, the splint maintains its shape quite nicely, though it does not provide as rigid an immobilization as does plaster.

Additional strips of material can be blended in with the splint to give additional stability, or mechanical techniques can be used to provide additional stability. The material is impervous to water and can be easily washed. It can also be remolded by heating. Localized changes in contour or position can be achieved by heating with a hot air blower, such as a hair dryer, or by heating with hot water. The material has a disadvantage in that it causes considerable perspiration and breaking out of the skin if applied directly to the skin without appropriate padding to protect the skin. Being completely impervious to water, it is nonabsorbent and calls for fabric interposition between it and the wound for absorption of secretions. The Orthoplast has the advantage that the splint can be washed completely clean and treated with disinfectants each time the dressing is reapplied; a high degree of cleanliness can be maintained with splints made of this material.

Recently, a variation of the plastic splint has been developed by Thermo-Mold Medical Products, and is marketed under the trade name of Warm 'N Form. This material is created from plastic but is covered with a fabric that

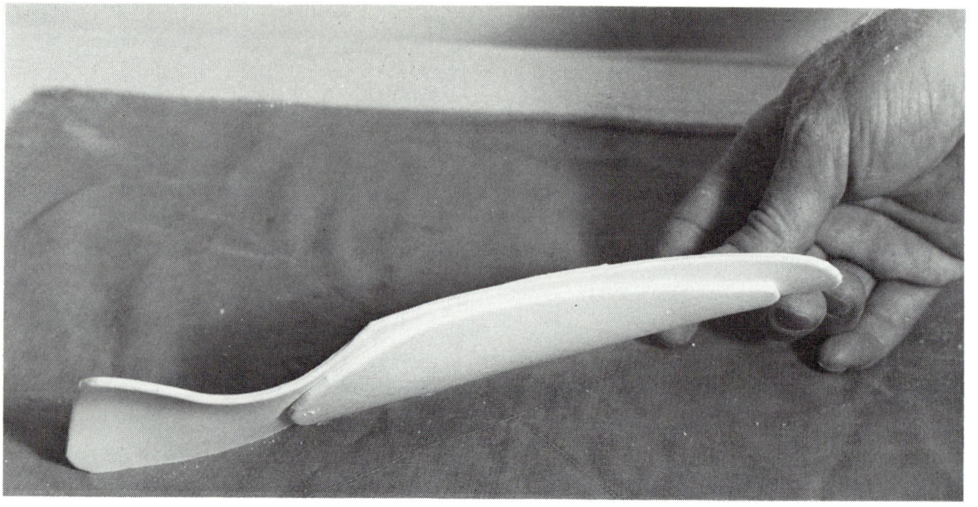

Fig. 6-4. An Orthoplast splint. The splint is cut to the appropriate size. Cutting is made much easier by first heating the material in hot water. The appropriate shape is then cut with scissors. Reinforcement in areas of particular stress is done by cutting a double layer and sticking them together with an agent such as acetone. The material is once again heated in hot water until it becomes quite pliable. It is applied over enough padding to prevent burning of the skin, and is held in place with an elastic bandage until it is cool enough to restore rigidity. The elastic bandage is then removed, and the splint is attached either by rewrapping the elastic bandage or attaching straps.

forms a permanent covering on the plastic. The fabric covering allows for a greater degree of acceptance by the skin since it is more absorbent and does not foster perspiration and associated skin rashes that develop with other splints. More recent designs of Warm 'N Form have included layers of plastic foam padding which improve the patient acceptability of this product. It is unnecessary to include different padding material between the splint and the extremity.

Warm 'N Form depends on the application of dry heat, since wet heat is contraindicated because of the fabric or foam backing. The material is heated on a hot plate designed to achieve the right temperature without burning the fabric backing. Once it has been heated, it can be cut very easily with special scissors and formed into almost any shape desired. Again, during the stage when it is still soft and pliable, it is molded around the extremity and made to follow the contour. As it cools, the material becomes quite rigid; it is the hardest of the plastic sheeting products in use today. It is virtually impossible to cut after it has cured, and it must be heated again to make it malleable enough to cut, even with the special scissors. The manufacturer recommends the incorporation of Velcro straps to hold the splint to the extremity. Special forms, such as those shown in Figure 6-5, are indicated for immobilization of the knee and elbow.

Once dry, the product has the favorable characteristics common to all the plastic sheeting splints—it is quite strong, resilient, light-weight, and x-ray penetratable. Warm 'N Form has the additional advantage of being less irritat-

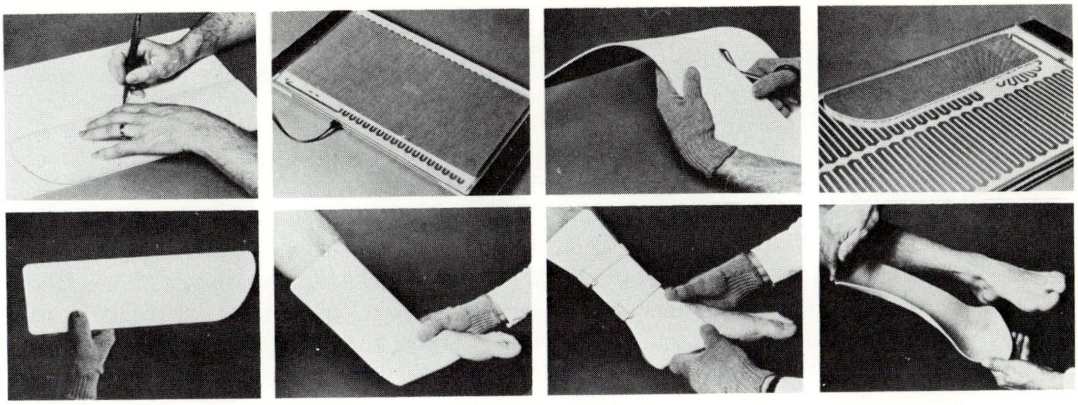

Fig. 6-5. The manufacture of splints from Warm 'N' Form. The material is extremely hard and resistant to cutting when cool. It is heated on a special electric warming plate provided for that purpose. When it is heated to the proper temperature, it is quite easily cut and shaped to the desired form. It is then applied to the extremity over a padding, since it can burn the skin if the skin is not protected. It is wrapped onto the extremity with an elastic bandage, or held in whatever manner desired, while it cools. The elastic bandages are then removed and the splint is attached to the extremity either by rewrapping with elastics or attaching straps or Velcro fasteners. Warm 'N Form cools much more rapidly than Orthoplast, and the working time is considerably shorter. Once cooling has been achieved, however, the material is much stronger than Orthoplast. (Courtesy of Thermo-Mold Medical Products, Inc.)

ing and more moisture absorbant than many of the plastic sheeting products without fabric backing.

Special Splints Also Can be Made of Metal. A popular form currently in use is the thin aluminum sheeting cut into appropriately sized splints and backed with an adherent plastic foam padding for use in the hand. The splints are quite malleable. The product is dispensed in long strips which can be cut to the appropriate length with ordinary bandage scissors. These splints are excellent for use in fingers, since they can be bent to form the desired contour but are rigid enough to prevent motion in the fingers. These splints are generally used on the palmar surface, though they can be folded over so that both a dorsal and volar component can be used to achieve greater strength and prevent motion in the treated finger. The fact that they are padded adequately with plastic foam adherent to the metal makes them even more adaptable for splinting the joints of the finger and the hand. Their malleability makes it possible to twist them so that the true contour of the hand can be followed faithfully. They are attached with strips of tape or with small rolls of elastic bandage for better support.

A bandage marketed by Johnson and Johnson under the trade name Coban has been found to be a very excellent material for attaching these splints to the finger or extremity. Coban is an elastic material similar to regular elastic bandages, except that it adheres to itself. It also is reusable. Its ability to adhere to itself makes it useful in the application of splints. It allows a very strong attachment of the splint to the extremity, and allows for removal of the splint when desired.

Other metal splinting materials are not malleable enough to be included here. They represent splints of the readymade variety.

Splints for Correction of Deformities

Along with their use for immobilization, splints also are used to provide correction of deformities. It has been previously noted that correction by casting is seldom possible; correction must be established before the cast is applied. This also is true of splints. It is seldom that a fracture that has not been properly aligned beforehand can be changed by splinting. However, corrections can be established by splints in soft-tissue deformities. It is in the treatment of these deformities, particularly of joints, that corrective splints show their greatest usefulness.

Where deformities have been corrected by surgery or by other means and are held by the splint, the correction is called a passive correction. It probably can be considered more of an immobilization than a true correction. There is a fine

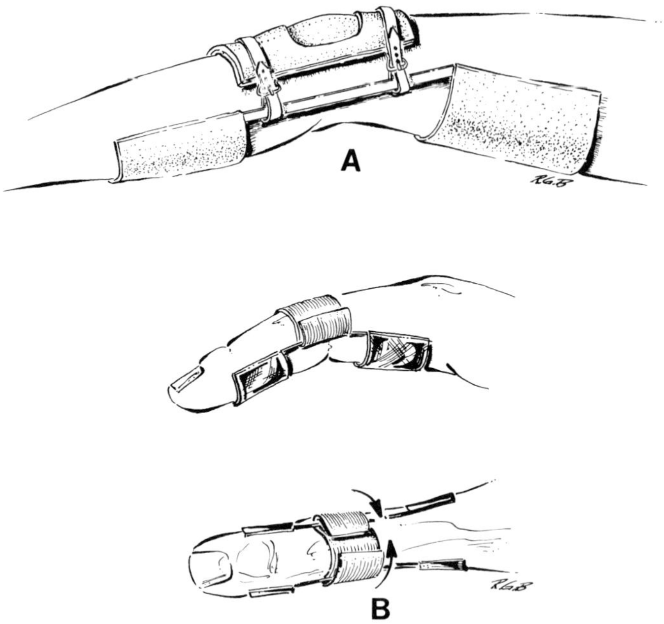

Fig. 6-6. Extension splints depend upon three-point pressure for their effectiveness. *(A)* An extensor splint on the knee. The metallic portion of the splint lies posteriorly, with bands on the thigh and the calf. Lying over the knee is a leather pad which is tightened with the knee in extension. It is not the purpose of this splint to dynamically correct a deformity; it merely maintains the maximum extension possible for a period of time. The splint is usually applied at night, after a warm bath, to stretch the knee out as far as possible. The extension is maintained during the night, which helps to stretch the structures holding the knee in flexion. If this is done nightly, the gradual increase in extension usually results in complete restoration of full extension. *(B)* An extensor splint on the finger. Again, dynamic correction is not sought, but rather the maintenance of maximum obtainable passive extension is applied over a period of time. Gradual increases in extension are obtained by passive stretching, and extension can be maintained once it has been achieved.

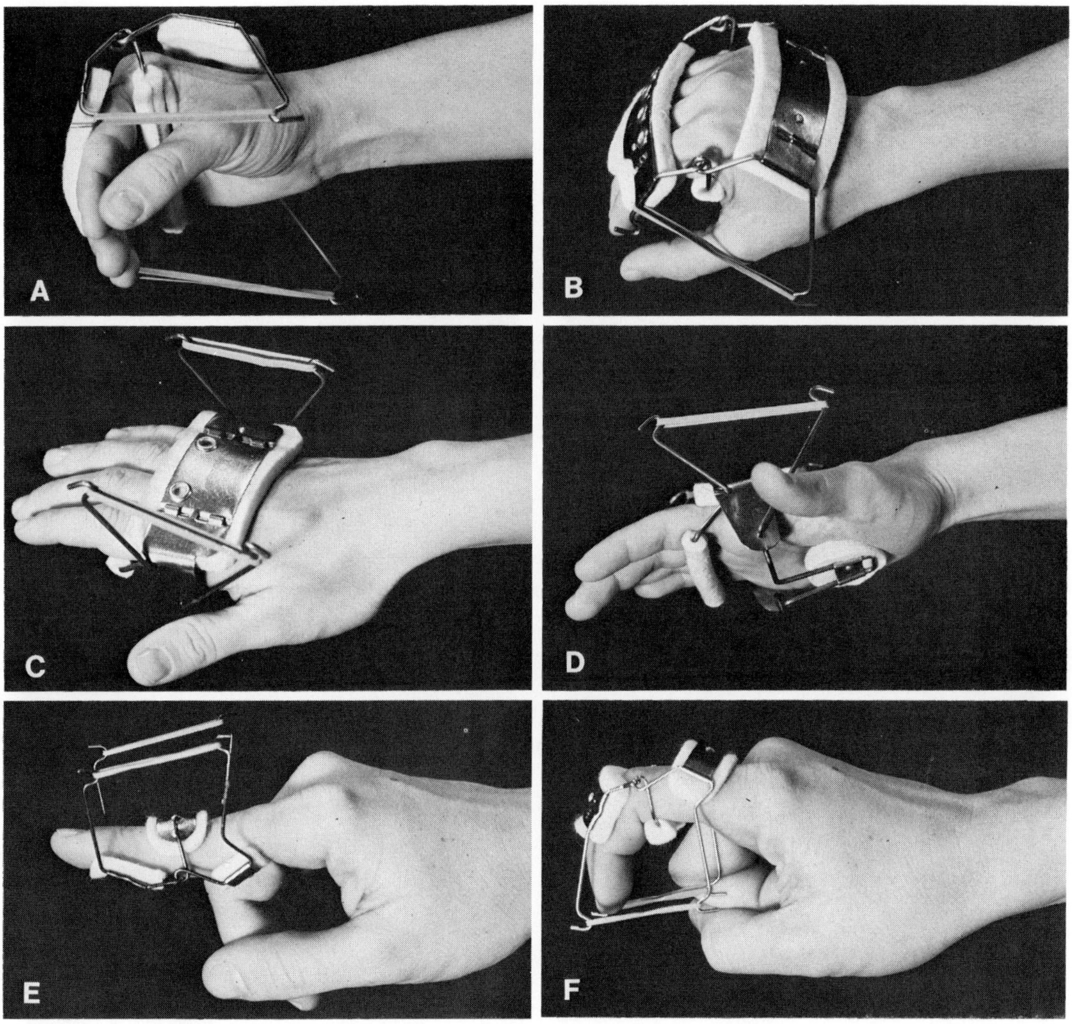

Fig. 6-7. (A and B) The Bunnell knuckle-bender splint is an example of the dynamic splint for continuous pressure to create flexion in the proximal joints of the fingers. The rubberband creates a positive force for pressing the joint into flexion. It should be noticed, however, that voluntary active extension of the joints against the traction can likewise be done, so that the splint not only acts as a dynamic force for flexion, but also acts as an exerciser for the extensor muscles of the fingers. *(C and D)* The Bunnell knuckle-extender splint has the exact opposite application of the knuckle-bender splint. The proximal joints of the fingers are forced into extension by the rubberband force, causing pressure in the palm and against the proximal phalanges. As is the case with the knuckle-bender splint, this may also be used as an exerciser for strengthening the finger flexors. *(E)* The Bunnell dynamic finger splint, showing extensor power being applied against the middle joint. *(F)* The same type of dynamic action in creating flexion of the middle joint. In both instances, as is the case with the knuckle bender and extender splints, the splint can be used for exercise against the rubberband traction, which may be as valuable a function as the dynamic power to correct a joint that is contracted either in flexion or extension.

line between the splint used for immobilization only and the splint used for passive correction. A good example of a passive correction splint is the extensor splint for flexion contractures of the knee. In Figure 6-6*A*, one can see that the splint acts as a passive force to correct the knee by stretching, and it acts to maintain the correction. An extension splint such as the one shown is used when flexion contractures of the knee have failed to regain complete extension following surgery. The patient is instructed to take a hot tub bath and soak the extremity prior to application of the splint. With the hot water, a gradual stretching of the joint is obtained; the splint is applied to help maintain the correction and, perhaps, to increase the correction slightly. The splint is worn as a night splint. It is the gradual increase of correction gained on each application that results in complete correction of the deformity.

Similar splints are applied to flexion contractures of the fingers (Fig. 6-6*B*). Three-point pressure is applied and gradually increased; a gradual correction of the deformity occurs as each degree of correction is gained and maintained.

Dynamic splints offer continuous or intermittent force that results in correction of deformities. An example of the dynamic correction of a flexion contracture of the finger is the Bunnell finger extender splint (Fig. 6-7*A*). The continuous application of force against the contracture results in gradual stretching of the contracture. By the same token, the force can be overcome by flexing the finger; as the finger is flexed and released, the gradual tugging on the joints afforded by the dynamic pressure of the rubber bands results in stretching of the contracture.

A similar appliance is the Oppenheimer splint pictured in Figure 6-8. This splint has a dynamic feature in the coil spring mechanism which holds the wrist in a cocked-up position. In cases of motor paralysis occasioned by loss of motor function in the radial nerve, the splint acts merely as a restraining

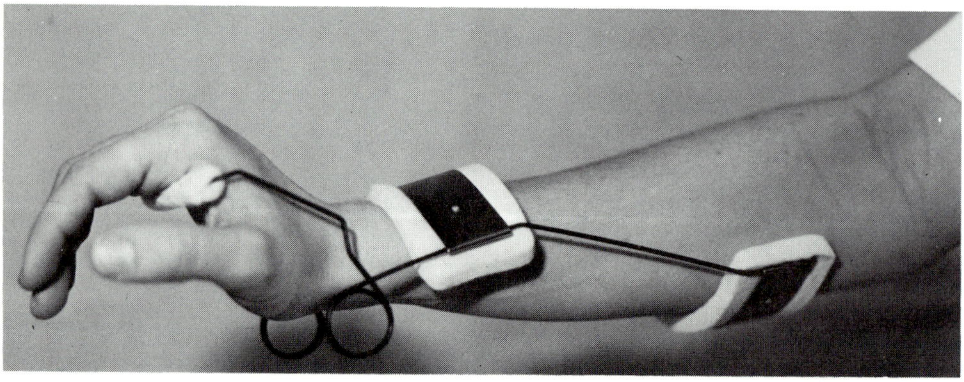

Fig. 6-8. The Oppenheimer splint is an excellent example of a dynamic splint used to create extension of the wrist. It is used basically in radial palsy, where the wrist extensors have lost motor function. It is occasionally also used to stretch flexion contractures of the wrist. It creates a continuous dynamic action in extension, but one which can be overcome by more powerful flexors, so that it acts as an exerciser for the flexor musculature of the wrist. This splint also has an out-rigger (not shown), which attaches by means of a leather sling with rubberband traction, to hold the thumb in extension when the extensor musculature of the thumb is paralyzed by radial palsy.

feature. It allows freer use of the wrist, since the spring mechanism can be overcome by the force of the flexors of the wrist pulling against it. This allows for a more nearly normal use. The Oppenheimer splint also can be used as a dynamic correction of flexion contractures of the wrist. It allows for a kinetic pull against the flexion contracture which is overcome periodically by use of the wrist flexors. When the flexors are released, a tugging occurs against the flexion contracture with gradual correction of the deformity.

OUTLINE OF PRINCIPLES

Many of these splints are recognizable models of standard corrective splints that have been used for years. It is not the purpose of this text to cover the myriad of splints and their specific uses. It is the purpose, however, to point out the fundamental principles of splinting and correction by splints. The practitioner who is able to fashion an original splint for a specific purpose, rather than one who uses a readymade, has grasped fully the concept of splinting. These basic principles, which should be kept in mind when creating a specific splint for a specific problem, are enumerated:

1. The corrective force, whether passive or dynamic, must be directly against the deformity itself with as little encroachment on the remainder of the extremity as possible.
2. For each correcting force there must be a counteracting force to help overcome the deformity. In the case of the Oppenheimer splint, a counterforce applied to the dorsum of the wrist holds the wrist in a position to allow extension of the hand on the fixed forearm. Were it not for this dorsal strap, which is applied over the distal portion of the forearm, the extensor power of the splint could not be realized in extending the wrist.
3. Dynamic correction splints are usually designed in such a manner that functioning muscles can overcome the dynamic correction periodically, giving the correcting force a greater function in periodically "tugging" at the fixed deformity.
4. Passive correction splints depend upon a gradual increase of pressure to afford correction. This is a passive pressure, however, and can be applied only to a moderate degree because of discomfort when maximum pressure is used.
5. In any passive or dynamic corrective splint, the lever arms must be designed to create a mechanical advantage sufficient to apply pressure at the fulcrum created at the point of deformity. One has only to remember the laws concerning levers to realize the effectiveness of this type of splinting. If the fulcrum is designed to apply maximum pressure of the lever arm system against the deformity, the splint should produce a satisfactory result.
6. The ability of corrective splints to overcome deformities depends upon the resilience of the tissue causing the deformity, the effect of growth, the ability of the surrounding tissue to accept the pressure required, and the accessibility of the deformity. These factors offer the following implications:
   A. The Resilience of Tissues. It is well known that old, well-developed, mature scar tissue is resistant to stretching. Once a scar has been allowed to mature, the chances of stretching it out by passive or dynamic

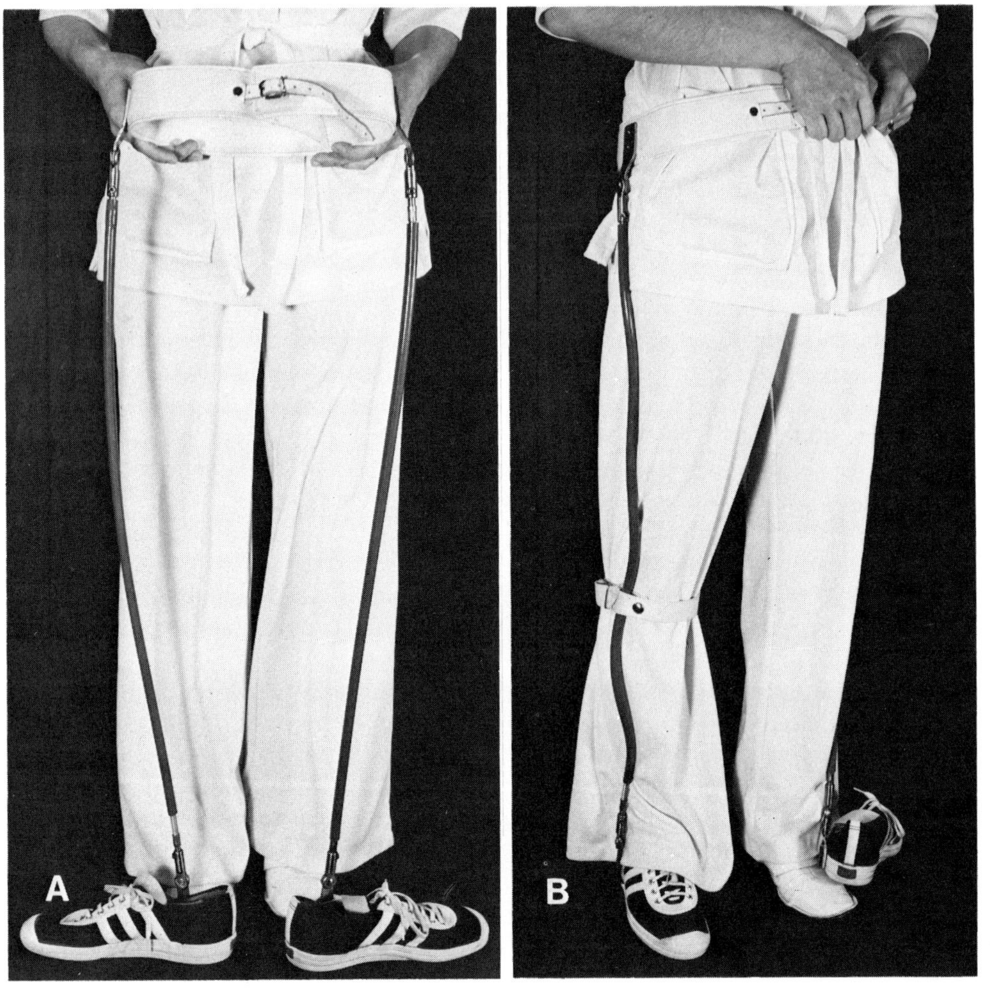

Fig. 6-9. The twister splint is an excellent mechanism for correcting deformities in the lower extremity. The twister cables are attached to a pelvic band and to the shoe. *(A)* The twisters hold the shoe in marked external rotation (or in internal rotation when necessary), but the power of the twister can be overcome by insertion of the foot in the shoe, *(B)*. Even when the foot is encased in the shoe, however, a continuous dynamic traction is applied to the foot, so that the entire extremity is forced into external rotation. This dynamic effect is useful both in internal rotation contractures of the hip and in instances of internal tibial torsion, wherein the continuous corrective force applied against the growing bone results in gradual correction by stimulating growth in the appropriate direction.

force are very limited. The use of corrective splints is of questionable value since one is attempting to overcome well-fixed scar tissue that has no elasticity and no chance for stretching. On the other hand, a young, immature scar is much more easily stretched. Scar tissue in younger individuals is more elastic than scar tissue in older individuals.

B. The Effect of Growth. The effect of growth cannot be overlooked. Continuous pressure along certain lines will result in growth changes caused

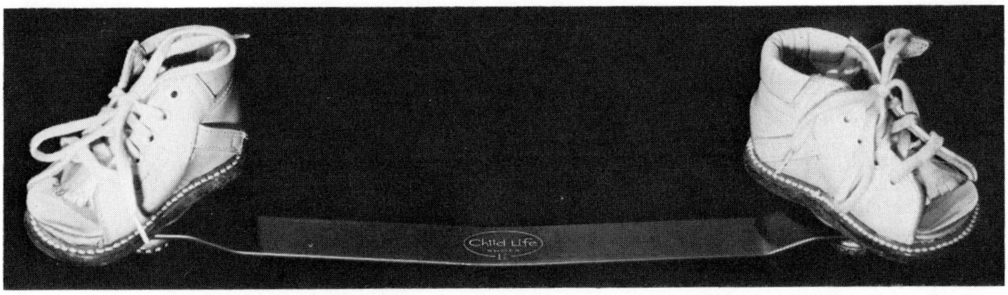

Fig. 6-10. The Denis-Browne splint. A passive corrective force is exerted, since the feet are inserted in the shoes which are held in the specific direction where correction is desired. The shoes have been set in external rotation, such as the position used for internal tibial torsion. While this constitutes a passive corrective force, it actually has more of a dynamic action, since the kicking action of the youngster results in continuous manipulation of the extremity, which hastens the corrective process. The splint, of course, can be set with the feet in internal rotation when external rotation deformities are to be corrected. Likewise, the angle of the bar can be bent so that inversion or eversion correction of the foot can be obtained simultaneously with the correction of torsional deformities.

by alterations in the mechanics of growth at the epiphyseal lines. Internal tibial torsion, treated in very young patients by twister cable splints with dynamic pressure for external rotation, corrects very rapidly because of the speed of growth occurring in the extremity (Fig. 6-9). By the same token, the use of the same splint in the older child, the juvenile, or the adult will be very disappointing. The growth potential in these individuals is either limited or absent and correction is not likely to take place. Correction in bone by corrective splints occurs only in the growing patient. The effect of any corrective splint on the long bone of a mature patient will not result in any appreciable change. Denis-Browne splints are also useful for correction of torsional deformities (Fig. 6-10). In the growing child, the development of soft-tissue contractures is much more likely to progress if the contracture occurs across epiphyseal lines that are still active. If the contracting band stays the same length and does not stretch while the epiphyseal centers continue to grow, the contracture will become more severe due to the tethering effect of the contracting band as growth occurs along the longitudinal axis of the bone. An example of the tethering effect is tightness of the heel cords which progresses in the rapidly growing child. The tight heel cord retains essentially the same length, but the longitudinal growth of the bone results in increased length of the extremity. The tethering effect of the heel cord results in a recurrence of the equinus deformity even though the heel cord itself has stayed essentially the same length.

C. The ability of the surrounding tissue to withstand the pressure required for correction of the deformity is often a limiting factor. In the case of the extensor splint for the knee, previously described, the patient will often complain of pain over the patella caused by pressure of the correcting strap, if it is applied too tightly. The limiting factor here, then, is the inability of the skin in the prepatellar area to withstand the pressure necessary to secure correction of the flexion contracture of the knee. The amount of force that can be used is dictated by the amount of pressure that can be tolerated at the point where the device presses upon the skin.

D. The accessibility of the contracture is likewise a limiting factor when applying correctional splints. The flexion contracture of the knee is quite accessible. An adequate splinting device can be arranged for correction of these deformities provided the flexion contracture is not so great as to preclude the application of a splint. If the flexion contracture is 45 degrees or less, an adequate splint can be made.

The middle joint of the finger, however, is sometimes not so accessible, particularly in the small individual who has a limited space available for a splint between the middle and proximal flexion creases of the finger. The length of lever arms available for a splint to stretch the middle joint are limited, and therefore the mechanical advantage for stretching this joint is limited. The accessibility of the joint and the ability to satisfactorily apply a splint to the deformity are of paramount importance when anticipating the amount of correction that can be obtained.

It is the purpose of this presentation to describe the fundamental principles of correction by splinting. It is hoped that these concepts will enable the reader to develop specific splints to serve specific purposes. There is a voluminous amount of literature that can be consulted concerning specific splinting techniques. The reader is referred to these for a more in-depth solution to any specific problem.

Index

Numerals in *italic* denote an illustration